CNOR® EXAM PREP
STUDY GUIDE

T0093439

CNOR® EXAM PREP STUDY GUIDE

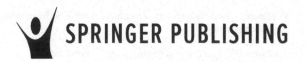

SPRINGER PUBLISHING

Copyright © 2024 Springer Publishing Company, LLC
All rights reserved.

No part of this publication may be reproduced, stored in a retrieval system, or transmitted in any form or by any means, electronic, mechanical, photo-copying, recording, or otherwise, without the prior permission of Springer Publishing Company, LLC, or authorization through payment of the appropriate fees to the Copyright Clearance Center, Inc., 222 Rosewood Drive, Danvers, MA 01923, 978-750-8400, fax 978-646-8600, info@copyright.com or at www.copyright.com.

Springer Publishing Company, LLC
11 West 42nd Street, New York, NY 10036
www.springerpub.com

Acquisitions Editor: Jaclyn Koshofer
Compositor: Exeter Premedia Services Private Ltd.

ISBN: 978-0-8261-6576-3
ebook ISBN: 978-0-8261-6626-5
DOI: 10.1891/9780826166265

23 24 25 26 / 5 4 3 2 1

The author and the publisher of this Work have made every effort to use sources believed to be reliable to provide information that is accurate and com-patible with the standards generally accepted at the time of publication. The author and publisher shall not be liable for any special, consequential, or exemplary damages resulting, in whole or in part, from the readers' use of, or reliance on, the information contained in this book. The publisher has no responsibility for the persistence or accuracy of URLs for external or third-party Internet websites referred to in this publication and does not guarantee that any content on such websites is, or will remain, accurate or appropriate.

CNOR® is a registered trademark of Competency & Credentialing Institute (CCI®). CCI® does not endorse this resource, nor does it have a proprietary relationship with Springer Publishing Company.

Library of Congress Control Number: 2023930024

Contact sales@springerpub.com to receive discount rates on bulk purchases.

Publisher's Note: New and used products purchased from third-party sellers are not guaranteed for quality, authenticity, or access to any included digital components.

Printed in the United States of America by Gasch Printing.

CONTENTS

PREFACE

This *Exam Prep Study Guide* was designed to be a high-speed review—a last-minute gut check before your exam day. We created this review to supplement your certification preparation studies. We encourage you to use it in conjunction with other study aids to ensure you are as prepared as possible for the exam.

This book follows the Competency & Credentialing Institute's most recent exam content outlines and uses a succinct, bulleted format to highlight what you need to know. The aim of this book is to help you solidify your retention of information in the month or so leading up to your exam. It is written by certified perioperative nurses who are familiar with the exam and the content you need to know. Special features appear throughout the book to call out important information, including:

- **Complications**: Problems that can arise with certain disease states or procedures
- **Nursing Pearls**: Additional patient care insights and strategies for knowledge retention
- **Alerts**: Need-to-know details on how to handle emergency situations or when to transfer care
- **Pop Quizzes**: Critical-thinking questions to test your ability to synthesize what you learned (answers are in the back of the book)
- **Two Full-Length Practice Tests**: One printed in the book, one online
- **Free One-Month Access to ExamPrepConnect**: The digital study platform that guides you confidently through your exam prep journey

We know life is busy. Being able to prepare for your exam efficiently and effectively is paramount, which is why we created this *Exam Prep Study Guide*. You have come to the right place as you continue on your path of professional growth and development. The stakes are high, and we want to help you succeed. Best of luck to you on your certification journey.

PASS GUARANTEE

If you use this resource to prepare for your exam and do not pass, you may return it for a refund of your full purchase price, excluding tax, shipping, and handling. To receive a refund, return your product along with a copy of your exam score report and original receipt showing purchase of new product (not used). Product must be returned and received within 180 days of the original purchase date. Refunds will be issued within 8 weeks from acceptance and approval. One offer per person and address. This offer is valid for U.S. residents only. Void where prohibited. To initiate a refund, please contact Customer Service at csexamprep@ springerpub.com.

1 GENERAL EXAMINATION INFORMATION

OVERVIEW

The CNOR® exam is administered by the Competency & Credentialing Institute (CCI®) to validate basic and advanced knowledge of nurses working in the preoperative, intraoperative, and postoperative phases of surgery. The exam serves as the foundation of established practice and the basis of comparison in future continuing education. Through the successful completion of the exam, the candidate will demonstrate competence in

- The nursing process through the incorporation of critical thinking to engage in safe patient care
- Perioperative nursing practice

CNOR CERTIFICATION

- The examination is open to all nurses meeting the licensure, continuing education, and experience criteria as set by CCI.
- Once the examination is completed and certification verified, the nurse may utilize CNOR credentialing as a professional designation.
- CCI has been certifying perioperative nurses for over four decades and has certified more than 40,000 perioperative nurses, surgical services managers, perioperative clinical nurse specialists, and other surgery-related nursing specialties worldwide.

ABOUT THE EXAMINATION

- The CNOR examination has 200 multiple choice questions and is 3.75 hr in length.
- Of the 200 multiple choice questions, 185 are scored, and 15 are pretest questions that are not scored.
- The examination blueprint covers the following topics: Pre/Postoperative Patient Assessment and Diagnosis; Individualized Plan of Care Development and Expected Outcome Identification; Management of Intraoperative Activities; Communication and Documentation; Infection Prevention and Control of Environment, Instrumentation, and Supplies; Emergency Situations; and Professional Accountabilities.
- The candidate must correctly answer at least 106 questions to pass the exam.
- Candidates have a 90-day window to take the examination starting the month after application is accepted.
- For information about examination accommodations, review the instructions in the testing handbook.

EXAM ELIGIBILITY

Candidates must meet the following minimum criteria to sit for the exam:

- Hold a license as an RN that is valid in the state or country where they work.
- Be currently working either full or part time in perioperative nursing, nursing education, research, or administration. ▶

EXAM ELIGIBILITY (*continued*)

- Have at least 2 years of experience in a clinical perioperative setting with at least 1,200 hr working experience as an intraoperative nurse.

HOW TO APPLY

- Candidates may apply by creating an account through CCI at https://www.cc-institute.org/cnor/apply; include work history, employer contact information, and supervisor contact information.
- Cost of the exam: $395.
- Timeline to test: Candidates may schedule the exam Monday through Sunday except for holidays. The 3-month testing window opens the month after candidates' applications have been approved. Once approved, candidates schedule the exam with a PSI testing center in their geographical area. PSI administers the exam. If there is difficulty in locating a PSI testing center, candidates may arrange to take their test via a remote proctor from locations of their choice.

HOW TO RECERTIFY

CNOR certification is active for 5 years. Candidates may recertify by meeting the following requirements:

- Confirm that the following credentials and work requirements are met: Hold an active CNOR credential and a current, unrestricted nursing license; work full or part time in perioperative nursing practice; and attest that a minimum of 500 hr have been worked in perioperative nursing, 250 of which must be in intraoperative care.
- Complete 300 required professional activity points during the 5-year accrual period.
- Submit a renewal application with fee through CCI.
- Candidates who have not completed the required professional activities can apply for a 1-year extension to earn points.

HOW TO CONTACT CCI

- Website: https://www.cc-institute.org
- Email: info@cc-institute.org
- Certification Administration: (303) 369-9566
- Fax: (303) 695-8464
- Mailing Address:

  Competency and Credentialing Institute
  400 Inverness Pkwy, Suite 265
  Englewood, CO 80112

RESOURCES

Competency & Credentialing Institute. (2022). *CNOR certification & recertification candidate handbook*. https://f.hubspotusercontent30.net/hubfs/2447632/Handbooks/CNOR%20Candidate%20Handbook.pdf

Competency & Credentialing Institute. (n.d.-a). *CNOR recertification*. https://www.cc-institute.org/cnor/certified-before-2018

Competency & Credentialing Institute. (n.d.-b). *CNOR recertification*. https://www.cc-institute.org/cnor/certified-after-2019

2 PRE- AND POSTOPERATIVE PATIENT ASSESSMENT AND DIAGNOSIS

OVERVIEW

- A preoperative patient assessment and diagnosis are performed to evaluate issues that pose a significant risk to the patient in the perioperative phase.
- A postoperative patient assessment is performed to evaluate the patient's overall condition and to assess the integrity of the skin and bony prominences immediately following surgical intervention.
- Evaluate for the expected outcomes and use the appropriate interventions if the goal is not achieved.
- *Note:* Throughout each phase of the perioperative experience, the nurse will perform duties using the ACE process: Assess, Confirm, and Evaluate and Ensure.

PREOPERATIVE ASSESSMENT

- The preoperative phase of the patient's surgical experience begins upon the decision to have surgery.
- The preoperative assessment is part of the preprocedure verification process, which is the first phase of the Universal Protocol. In this phase of perioperative care, a preprocedure verification is performed to prevent wrong-person, wrong-site, and wrong-procedure occurrences. The preoperative assessment serves the following functions: Identifying patients who are at higher risk for surgical complication associated with the following factors: Promoting patient safety throughout the perioperative period; providing the surgical team with the necessary information concerning the patient's baseline health status, which is then used to compare intraoperatively and postoperatively and assess for anomalies; and uncovering comorbidities and other health risks that might contribute to intraoperative complications. Some of the primary comorbidities that contribute to complications include cardiovascular disease, obstructive sleep apnea (OSA), and reactive airway disease (asthma, chronic obstructive pulmonary disease [COPD]).

Assess

- Patient record review: accurate height and weight, allergies and adverse drug reactions, chief complaint, and history of present illness
- Past medical history: comorbidities such as diabetes mellitus (DM), coronary artery disease (CAD), COPD, chronic kidney disease (CKD), OSA, clotting disorder, and so on; presence of existing implants; presence of sensory impairment associated with hearing; presence of visual impairment; presence of impairment associated with cognitive function; and preexisting medical conditions that can increase the risk of fluid and electrolyte imbalance
- Past surgical history (e.g., prior surgeries, mastectomy, implanted stimulators)
- Medication review: medication reconciliation present on the chart; report of last medications taken and time taken (beta-blockers within the last 24 hr, administration of prophylactic antibiotics, antimicrobial bathing, etc.); and that all aspects of the medication reconciliation are complete
- Family history: report of significant family history (history of heart disease, clotting disorder, etc.) ►

Assess (*continued*)

- Social history: alcohol use or history of alcohol use, diet and diet restrictions associated with preexisting conditions, illicit drug use or history of illicit drug use, and exercise routine
- Cultural assessment: evaluation of the patient's cultural background, education, and cultural needs; examination and accommodation of patient's religious beliefs; and use of translation services if needed
- Functional assessment: age-specific psychosocial assessment, basic evaluation of the patient's physical strength and pulses, complications with range of motion that may limit procedural positioning needs, patient's ability to perform activities of daily living (ADLs), and sensory deficits and neurologic function
- Review of systems: review of systems conducted by the preadmission testing office and anesthesia personnel
- Physical examination: patient's pain level and patient's skin
- Laboratory and diagnostic tests will be ordered by either the surgeon, anesthesiologist, or both depending on the patient's surgery and comorbidities

[ ]   **NURSING PEARL**

SAMPLE Mnemonic

Rothrock identified the mnemonic SAMPLE as a quick guide to gather the pertinent history. In emergent situations, this may be gathered after the surgical intervention has begun.

- **S**ymptoms
- **A**llergies
- **M**edications
- **P**ast medical history
- **L**ast oral intake
- **E**vents or Environment that led to the accident or injury

---

[UNFOLDING SCENARIO 2.1A]

A 54-year-old female patient is scheduled for hysteroscopy with dilation and curettage. Patient education was provided related to lithotomy positioning and expectations after the procedure. Piercings have been removed. The patient denies alcohol or drug use and is a nonsmoker. The patient has been nothing by mouth (NPO) since midnight and took only lisinopril 10 mg with a sip of water this morning. The patient reports having lumbar fusion and low back pain. The patient weighs 152 lb. and is 5 ft. 4 in. tall. Warm blankets have been placed on the patient.

Question

What other aspects of the preoperative assessment are necessary?

Confirm

- Informed consent: The patient has been informed of the description of the procedure and alternative therapies, explanation of risks associated with the procedure, explanation that the patient has the right to refuse treatment or withdraw consent, name and qualifications of the person(s) performing the procedure, and underlying disease process and natural course. The patient has no questions related to the planned procedure. The patient (or their representative) has signed (on paper or electronically) verifying consent to the surgical procedure. ▶

[ ]   **ALERT!**

The perioperative nurse may serve as the witness to consent. It is the nurse's function to ensure that the patient can verbalize understanding of the procedure to be performed and has no questions. All documents (such as the surgical consent, advance directive, and do-not-resuscitate order) must be fully executed before the patient can be taken to the surgical suite for the procedure.

Confirm (*continued*)

- Patient identification: If the patient is suffering from cognitive impairment or cannot verbalize their name and date of birth, the patient's identity verification process should be performed per the organization's policy and procedure. In some cases, the patient's medical record number will also be checked if the organization is utilizing barcode medication scanning.
- Code status per Association of periOperative Registered Nurses (AORN): Confirm that the advance directive or do-not-resuscitate order (where applicable) is complete and present on the patient's chart.
- Correct procedure and site marking: Confirm the site is marked with a marker that will withstand the prep solution of choice so that the mark is apparent and visible to all team members after preparation. Ensure that all consents are in the chart and that they are signed.
- Surgical environment: Confirm the OR is stocked with the following basic room contents—anesthesia machine and supplies, biohazard receptacle, electrical surgical unit (ESU), instrument table, kick bucket, linen hamper, mayo stand, other supplies and equipment as required by the procedure, OR bed or table, prep table, sharps container, suction apparatus and supplies, and a trash bin. Also ensure the cleanliness of the surgical suite.
- Specimen management needs: Collaborate with the surgeon to address the prospective specimen to be collected, handling, and disposition; need for photography equipment (e.g., Mohs procedures); and specimen collection equipment.

Evaluate and Ensure

- Ensure there are no barriers to completing a perioperative assessment, such as emergent situations. NPO status (or lack thereof) can cause surgery cancellation or delay. Language barriers can cause a delay in the procedure due to a need to access an interpreter. Cultural barriers can create communication barriers and delay the procedure. Cognitive impairment can create communication barriers. Missing test results, history, and physical assessment can create delays in the scheduled procedure time.
- Ensure that the patient has received adequate education. Answer any last-minute questions and ensure the patient and family member(s) verbalize understanding of the procedure. Patient education must be tailored to the patient's age, readiness to learn, level of learning, and culture. Teaching materials should be provided to patients and their family members and written at the patient's level of literacy.
- Ensure family/contact presence. Make sure there is an up-to-date contact number in the chart so that the surgeon may update the appropriate family member/friend intra- and postop.
- Ensure the following last-minute considerations: A urinary catheter has been placed, if indicated; active type and screen, so appropriate blood products have been typed and crossed and are available in the blood bank; all personal articles have been removed; any diagnostic tests/lab results are available in the chart; normothermia measures (blankets, forced-air warmers) are in place for perioperative and postoperative implementation; special equipment is available; and the patient has been NPO since midnight.

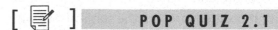

POP QUIZ 2.1

A 56-year-old male is admitted through the preoperative patient holding area for left shoulder arthroplasty. The nurse is performing the preoperative assessment and notices that the surgical site has not been marked. The anesthesiologist is set up to perform a scalene nerve block. What should the nurse do?

[**UNFOLDING SCENARIO 2.1B**]

> After the patient has been intubated and anesthesia has commenced, the patient is positioned on the OR table and legs placed in the padded stirrups. The safety belt is securely strapped across the patient's abdomen at the request of the surgeon. The sterile draping and surgical prep are applied by the scrub technician.
>
> **Question**
>
> *What is the circulating nurse's next course of action?*

INTRAOPERATIVE ASSESSMENT AND UNIVERSAL PROTOCOL

- The intraoperative phase begins when the patient is transferred onto the OR bed or table.
- The perioperative nurse uses the nursing process to guide nursing practice and enhance perioperative assessment.
- The Universal Protocol starts in the preoperative phase; however, it is centered around the time-out process, which occurs in the intraoperative phase.
- The Universal Protocol is a safety practice developed by The Joint Commission (TJC) that begins in the preoperative phase and continues during the intraoperative phase. It consists of conducting a preprocedure verification process, marking the surgical site as appropriate, and performing the time-out.

Assess

- Preprocedure verification process: Verify the correct procedure, patient, and site (involve the patient when necessary); identify the items needed for the procedure (implants, equipment, instrumentation, medications, personnel); and utilize a standardized list to verify the availability of items needed for the procedure.

[ ]   **ALERT!**

TJC identified that in the case of an unconscious patient, the nurse should follow the policy established by the facility related to the identification process. Further, TJC also identified that the facility may use temporary names until family members identify the patient.

- Patient setup: Place the patient on the OR table; assist anesthesia personnel with proper connection of monitoring; the anesthesia personnel may intubate the patient, place a central line, and place an arterial line; set up medication, to include priming of appropriate medications and intravenous (IV) pump setup, having emergency medications prepared, and so on; maintain patient privacy; clear pathway around the sterile field; insert urinary catheter (if not already done during preop); position patient for specific procedure and ensure patient is properly secured with appropriate safety straps; clip hair at the surgical site if ordered; prepare the surgical site with chlorhexidine or other solution as ordered.
- Type of wound closure to be performed: *Primary intention*—characterized by wounds created under sterile conditions, with minimal tissue destruction present with edges of wounds approximated. *Secondary intention*—characterized by chronic, dirty, or infected wounds not closed and allowed to heal through granulation. *Delayed primary closure or tertiary intention*—characterized by wounds requiring debridement and delayed healing of 3 days or more after injury or surgical intervention.
- Wound management consists of several approaches. *Debridement*—removal of devitalized tissue from the wound through sharp excision, mechanical irrigation, enzymatic agents, or biologic methods. *Hydrotherapy*—used in the OR and is referred to as pulsatile lavage. *Hydrosurgery*—performed using pressurized irrigation and localized vacuum to remove devitalized tissue. *Hyperbaric oxygenation*—use of a hyperbaric chamber to increase oxygenation to the wound. The chamber can also encourage cellular regeneration for chronic wounds. *Negative-pressure wound therapy*—use of a vacuum-assisted closure device, drainage sponge, and occlusive dressing for the long-term management of chronic or nonhealing wounds. ▶

Assess (*continued*)

- Risk factors: Blood loss is likely during a surgical event; arthroscopic surgery requires introduction of an increased amount of normal saline to the surgical site for visualization (fluid can leech into the surrounding tissues and vasculature); abdominal surgery involving the bowel or pancreas can cause third spacing; gastrointestinal surgery can cause bowel preparation (associated presentation of dehydration); neurosurgery causes dysregulation of antidiuretic hormone and hyponatremia; vaginal hysteroscopy requires introduction of sterile fluids to improve visualization of the pelvic organs (fluids can leech into the surrounding tissues and vasculature), and fluid overload or excessive loss can occur through cell damage related to manipulation during surgery, drains, nasogastric tube suctioning, prolonged surgery time, and stoma leakage.
- Assess the placement of dispersive electrode grounding pad (Bovie pad); protect the patient from electric shock or burns by placing a dispersive electrode grounding pad on the patient; avoid placement of the grounding pad on hair, bony prominences, dry skin, or adipose tissue; place the adhesive side of the grounding pad on an area of the body that is as far away from an implanted pacemaker or implantable cardioverter-defibrillator (ICD) as possible, flush to the skin and not tented, not over any metal implants or prosthesis (e.g., hip implants, knee implants, rods), on an area that has muscle mass and vascularity, and opposite of the surgical site; plug the pad into the ESU, and position the ESU on the same side as the primary surgeon where the settings can be visualized; and confirm the current type to be used with the surgeon.

Special Considerations

- Pediatric patient assessment considerations include airway and lungs, cardiovascular, fluid management, metabolism, temperature regulation, and skin and prep solutions.
- Trauma surgery and advanced trauma life support (ATLS) assessment considerations: Upon transfer of the patient from the emergency department to the perioperative suite, the provider should assess the patient's airway, respiratory function, and circulation; assess the level of neurologic disability; and examine the extent of the injuries and thermoregulation of the patient. After the preliminary assessment is complete, a secondary assessment is performed.

Confirm

- Conduct the time-out immediately before the invasive procedure or before the incision is made. All team members must agree on the correct patient identity, site, procedure to be done, administration of antibiotics (if required), and confirmation that all items needed for surgery are present in the surgical suite. ▶

[⊕] NURSING PEARL

Association of periOperative Registered Nurses Wound Classification

- *Class I:* Class I includes clean wounds that are not infected and show no signs of inflammation.
- *Class II:* Clean-contaminated wounds are associated with the respiratory, alimentary, or genitourinary tract where no infection or break in aseptic technique is present.
- *Class III:* Contaminated wounds are related to accidents, penetrating trauma, fractures, and operations with multiple breaks in aseptic technique. Some signs of infection and gross spillage of infectious material may be present.
- *Class IV:* Dirty or infected wounds are traumatic and contain retained devitalized tissue. The wound contains infectious material.

[⚡] ALERT!

TJC Universal Protocol Standard UP0101: Element of Performance 1 requires that a preprocedure process is performed to verify the correct procedure, patient, and site. The patient should be involved in this process whenever possible.

[⚡] ALERT!

AORN recommends that the perioperative nurse functions as a patient advocate and communicates with all members of the surgical team and other nursing personnel to ensure that all the components of the universal protocol have been addressed.

Confirm (*continued*)

- Verify correct site marking, as noted preoperatively.
- Confirm patient safety measures have been performed (e.g., placement of the safety strap).
- Confirm combined roles/duties of the scrub and circulating nurse have been performed. Ensure that any contamination encountered during the procedure has been confined and contained. Perform a surgical count at the beginning and the end of the procedure, as well as any time a count is called for during the procedure. Ensure that all surgical team members are aware that a surgical count has taken place and the result of said count is communicated. All activity must cease in the event that there is an incorrect count. Work collaboratively with the surgeon and anesthesia team to promote positive patient outcomes.
- Confirm specific roles/duties of the scrub nurse have been performed. The scrub nurse collaborates with the circulating nurse to set up the OR suite for the procedure; collaborates with the surgeon related to the procedural needs; drapes all tables, stands, and sterile field; ensures ESU pencil or other apparatus is safely stowed when not in use and ensures tip is kept clean; ensures that sterility of the surgical field is maintained, instrumentation is passed in safe manner, all sharps and sponges are accounted for, and patient safety is preserved; establishes baseline counts for all sponges, sharps, and other countable materials used; gowns members of the surgical team; labels medications; maintains sterile technique during the procedure; manages sterile field and breaches in technique; passes all cords off in one direction if possible; prepares hemostatic agents as required for the procedure; prepares sterile instruments and supplies; prevents retained foreign objects in patient; positions all tables, stands, and equipment after draping; reconciles count; safely handles and manages all sharps, sutures, and other related closure materials; sets up drains and dressings; and validates medications dispensed to the sterile field.

[ ]   ALERT!

There are three types of hazards in the OR environment:

- *Biologic:* Pathogenic organisms, infectious waste, needlesticks or cuts, and latex sensitivity
- *Chemical:* Anesthesia gas exposure, toxic fumes or electrocautery plume, cytotoxic drugs, and cleaning agents
- *Physical:* Falls, noise, irradiation, and fire

- Confirm specific roles/duties of the circulating nurse have been completed. The circulating nurse applies the dispersive electrode pad; assists with OR suite preparation; assists with transfer of patient; assists anesthesia personnel during induction and intraoperatively (as needed); checks all case items/equipment and compares against the physician preference list; charges patient for only items used; collaborates with all surgical team members to promote patient outcomes and safety; coordinates connection of equipment adjacent to sterile field; documents all patient care and interventions according to facility policy and procedure; ensures the pathway around sterile field perimeter is clear and safety hazards have been addressed (cords, equipment, foot pedals, etc.); initiates time-out; inspects all package integrity; maintains accountability for instruments, sponges, sharps, and specimen handling; monitors for breaches in technique; obtains and dispenses solutions to sterile field using continuous motion to avoid aerosolization; opens all sterile supplies with assistance from surgical scrub person or other facilitating nurse; performs ongoing evaluation of patient's fluid output and notes/advises surgical team of blood loss and fluid amounts; performs skin asepsis as directed by surgeon or ensures that skin asepsis is performed correctly; positions OR bed corresponding to overhead lighting; prepares medications for dispensation to field; pretests equipment; promotes a culture of safety and advocates for patient; performs handoff reporting to recovery room nurse; tests overhead lights, suction, and other equipment as appropriate; and validates implants.

[UNFOLDING SCENARIO 2.1C]

After the patient has been intubated and anesthesia commenced, the patient is positioned on the OR table with their torso, neck, and head in the supine position and legs placed in the padded stirrups. The sterile draping is about to be applied when the circulating nurse notices that the safety strap is laying on the floor. The anesthesia personnel confirm that the arm straps are secure on both arms.

Question

What is the circulating nurse's next course of action?

Evaluate and Ensure

- Instrument sterility using Spaulding classification system: Critical—must be sterile and will enter tissue or vascular system (instruments, cutting endoscopic accessories, needles). Semi-critical—should be sterile but high-level disinfection acceptable according to manufacturer's instructions for use (IFUs) (anesthesia equipment, endoscopes). Noncritical—intermediate-to low-level disinfection or cleaning required (OR beds and linens, patient care items). Sterility maintained using aseptic technique when dispensing materials and instruments to sterile field.
- Surgical environment safety check preventing slips and falls: Arrange equipment and supplies to promote an unobstructed path, limit traffic and provide clear pathways in the suite, post signage where wet floors are present, rapidly clean up spills and debris, reduce clutter and cords on the floor, and wear slip-resistant footwear and shoe covers.
- Intraoperative complication evaluation: deep vein thrombosis (DVT) symptoms (most commonly seen postoperatively); respiratory complications; pain sensation, which can be noted by hypertension and tachycardia; bruising; red or darkened skin; swollen veins; warmth and tenderness at the site; hematoma; hypovolemia; hypervolemia; vital sign (VS) changes dependent on clinical status, specific surgery performed, and presence of comorbidities may occur intraoperatively but is medically managed by anesthesia team collaboration with surgeon.

ALERT!

TJC Universal Protocol Standard UP0101: Element of Performance 2 requires that relevant documentation and all labeled diagnostic and radiology test results are appropriately displayed in the surgical suite. Additionally, this element of performance requires that blood products, implantable materials and devices, and other special equipment are available for the procedure.

POP QUIZ 2.2

A 67-year-old female is admitted through the preoperative patient holding area for a right knee arthroscopy. A right femoral nerve block was administered by anesthesia personnel in the preoperative holding area to save time. While moving the patient from the stretcher to the surgical table, the nurse notices that the surgeon marked the left knee. What is the most appropriate action for the circulating nurse?

POSTOPERATIVE ASSESSMENT

- The postoperative assessment is performed, in varying degrees, by the entire surgical team.
- Postoperatively, the patient is admitted either to the postanesthesia care unit or the ICU, depending upon the patient's acuity.

Assess

■ Perform a postop assessment: Assess vital signs frequently depending on type of anesthesia needed (e.g., local only), clinical status, and institutional guidelines; evaluate the patient's pain level and administer pharmacologic agents as ordered; assess for skin integrity; if the wound is uncovered, assess the wound closure (closed and intact, or open for healing by secondary intention); and evaluate for wound healing complications.

■ Consider during the recovery period: Can the patient have food and drink if recovering well postop? Is the patient waking up appropriately from anesthesia? If the patient is intubated, are they reversed (if paralyzed)? Does the surgeon want postop labs sent? Does the patient need blood products?

■ Some facilities may require frequent assessments including the use of the Aldrete scoring system (measurement of recovery after anesthesia). Use the appropriate postop protocol for the institution.

Confirm

■ Actions to occur at the end of the procedure: Provide assistance to anesthesia personnel during the extubation of the patient, if indicated; ensure that dressings are applied by appropriate scrubbed staff (nurse, technician, registered nurse first assistant [RNFA], physician assistant [PA], NP, surgeon); ensure the patient is safely repositioned to a supine position with assistance; ensure the transfer of the patient to the stretcher or bed is performed by at least four people.

■ Specimen procurement and confirmation: Specimen procurement and confirmation will be completed by the circulating nurse and scrub personnel through assisting the surgeon in receiving verbal confirmation of the diagnosis or specimen-related details with the pathologist (related to specimens sent for frozen section), labelling accurately, minimizing the risk of specimen compromise through careful transfer from the sterile field, reducing the number of people involved in the specimen handling process, using a dedicated space for specimen management on and off the sterile field, verifying the patient identification and specimen identification on the label with the read-back method to review specimen names and disposition has been performed, confirming the procedure performed is recorded in the patient's health record, and noting that deviations from the primary scheduled procedure can occur and are related to complications experienced during surgery.

■ Surgical counts: Ensure that surgical counts (sponges, instruments, sharps, and any other materials) have been completed and the surgical team has been made aware of any discrepancies. If there is a discrepancy noted, follow the institutional policy for discrepancy resolution and documentation. Ensure that normothermia is maintained by placing warm blankets (or forced-air warming) on the patient immediately following the application of dressings and maintain the position of drains (if used). Ensure drains that have not moved are appropriately secured, if applicable.

■ Cleaning with Food and Drug Administration (FDA)-approved disinfectant at the end of the procedure: Place biohazardous material in the appropriate receptacle following the procedure, dispose of sharps in the appropriate containers, and dispose solutions and suction container contents according to the facility policy.

[⊕]   **NURSING PEARL**

Wound Healing Phases

• *Inflammatory*: This phase lasts 0 to 3 days with redness, edema, and phagocytosis occurring.

• *Proliferation*: This phase lasts 4 to 24 days with granulation and epithelial tissue forming.

• *Maturation*: This phase lasts 24 days to 1 year with scar formation and contracture of tissue forming.

[▨]   **POP QUIZ 2.3**

A 77-year-old male is admitted through the preoperative patient holding area for a right total knee arthroplasty. The patient sustained blood loss associated with injury to the popliteal artery. The patient will likely need a blood transfusion postoperatively. To promote continuity of care, what should the circulating nurse report to the post-anesthesia care unit (PACU) nurse?

Evaluate and Ensure

- Ensure the following actions have occurred at the end of the procedure: All contaminated items are removed; drains are appropriately secured, draining, and patent; patient is positioned back on bed safely; family has been updated; nonradiopaque sponges are removed; and normothermia is maintained.
- Evaluation of the patient's clinical status: Extubation readiness (per surgeon and anesthesia personnel); and recovery need evaluation of the patient (PACU or ICU) based on patient's clinical status and recommendations of surgery and anesthesia team.
- Effective communication and handoff reporting to receiving unit; postop report process specific to facility.

[UNFOLDING SCENARIO 2.1D]

After the procedure, the circulating nurse notices that hysteroscopy irrigation has leaked on the floor and is not part of the output volume collected in the suction canister. While repositioning the patient from lithotomy to supine position with assistance from the scrub technician, the circulating nurse notices that the patient's legs are edematous. The surgeon has already left the room.

Question

What is the circulating nurse's next course of action?

[UNFOLDING SCENARIO 2.2A]

A 58-year-old female patient is scheduled for a laparoscopic low anterior bowel resection related to a cancerous tumor found on a CT scan. The following are the preoperative assessment findings.

- Paperwork
  - All paperwork (anesthesia consent, surgical consent, history and physical, and associated laboratory and diagnostic workup) are present.
- VS
  - *Initial VS are EKG:* Normal sinus rhythm (NSR), blood pressure (BP) 110/60, heart rate (HR) 72, 16; SpO_2 100%.
  - The patient is intubated with a 7.0-mm endotracheal tube (ETT) without difficulty. Preoperatively, a 20-gauge IV is placed in the right antecubital fossa. The cystic artery is cut, and the laparoscopic bowel resection is emergently converted to an open procedure. An additional 16-gauge IV has been placed in the left antecubital fossa; both IVs are wide open with fluids being administered. An esophageal temperature probe has been inserted. An arterial line has been inserted into the right radial artery. Current fluid volume deficit indicators are thready pulse, decreased venous filling, and decreased cardiac output.

(continued)

[UNFOLDING SCENARIO 2.2A] (continued)

- ▪ Lab values show two critical issues. Here are the baseline laboratory results:
  - ○ *White blood cell (WBC) 9.7 103/μL Reference range:* 4.0 to 11.0
  - ○ *Red blood cell (RBC) 5.5 106/μL Reference range:* 4.6 to 6.2
  - ○ *Hemoglobin (HgB) 11.0 g/dL Reference range:* 12.0 to 15.0
  - ○ *Hematocrit (HCT) 34 % Reference range:* 36 to 46
  - ○ *Platelets (PLT) 410 cells/μL Reference range:* 140 to 450
  - ○ No pregnancy test performed due to patient hysterectomy at age 50 years
- ▪ History and physical
  - ○ Patient education was provided related to the possibility of repositioning during the procedure to lithotomy to improve access and associated with the surgeon's surgical approach.
  - ○ Piercings have been removed.
  - ○ The patient denies alcohol or drug use and is a nonsmoker.
  - ○ The patient is married and has two children.
  - ○ The patient is a Jehovah's Witness and has declined to sign the blood consent.
  - ○ The patient has been NPO since midnight and took only metoprolol 25 mg with a sip of water in the morning.
  - ○ The patient reported a scar associated with a cesarean section 20 years ago.
  - ○ The patient weighs 145 lb. and is 5 ft. 4 in. tall.

Question

What other aspects of the assessment are necessary?

[UNFOLDING SCENARIO 2.2B]

The surgeon begins to perform the bowel resection and notices that there are multiple adhesions wrapped around the area of the bowel to be resected. The surgeon begins to perform soft dissection to gently remove the adhesions when the bowel perforates. Gross fecal spillage from the intestine begins to fill the abdominal cavity, and the patient begins to hemorrhage.

Question

What is the circulating nurse's next course of action both off and on the sterile field?

[UNFOLDING SCENARIO 2.2C]

The anesthesiologist alerts the surgeon that the patient has become tachycardic and asks how much blood was lost. The circulating nurse verbalizes to the team the volume of blood and fluid collected in the suction canister (3L). The circulator reminds the team that the patient is a Jehovah's Witness and refused to sign the blood consent, even though patient education from the surgeon and anesthesiologist was provided.

The surgeon successfully stops the bleeding and resects the bowel. The surgical cavity is irrigated. The anesthesiologist pages the chief of anesthesia to take over for the anesthesiologist of record, who left to consult the patient's family. The anesthesiologist of record returns to the room stating that he received consent for blood products and transfusion from the patient's husband, who is listed as the medical decision-maker in the living will on the chart.

Question

What is the circulating nurse's next course of action related to the transfusion?

RESOURCES

Association of periOperative Registered Nurses. (2016). *AORN Perioperative efficiency toolkit*. https://www.aorn.org/-/media/aorn/guidelines/tool-kits/perioperative-efficiency/aorn-perioperative-efficiency-tool-kit-webinar.pdf?la=en

Association of periOperative Registered Nurses. (2019). *Guideline essentials: Key takeaways. Team communication*. https://www.aorn.org/essentials/team-communication

Association of periOperative Registered Nurses. (2021). *Position statement: Preventing wrong-patient, wrong-site, wrong-procedure events*. https://www.aorn.org/-/media/aorn/guidelines/position-statements/posstat-wrong-site-0302.pdf

Caple, C. R. B. M., & Kornusky, J. R. M. (2018). *Preoperative assessment: Performing*. CINAHL nursing guide. EBSCO.

The Joint Commission. (n.d.). *The Universal Protocol*. https://www.jointcommission.org/standards/universal-protocol

The Joint Commission. (2022, August 29). *What are the key elements organizations need to understand regarding the use of two patient identifiers prior to providing care, treatment or services?* https://www.jointcommission.org/standards/standard-faqs/home-care/national-patient-safety-goals-npsg/000001545

Phillips, N., & Hornacky, A. (2021). *Berry and Kohn's operating room technique* (14th ed.). Elsevier.

Rothrock, J. C., & McEwen, D. R. (Eds.). (2019). *Alexander's care of the patient in surgery* (16th ed.). Elsevier.

3 INDIVIDUALIZED PLANS OF CARE AND EXPECTED OUTCOMES

OVERVIEW

- A perioperative nurse should develop comprehensive plans of care spanning the preoperative, intraoperative, and postoperative phases of the surgical experience using an evidence-based practice (EBP) approach that follows the nursing process and incorporates perioperative nursing data set (PNDS) standard nursing language.
- Each patient's plan of care is individualized based on patient-specific assessment data. This ensures the best patient outcomes and highest quality care.
- The perioperative nurse uses North American Nursing Diagnosis Association (NANDA) guidance to formulate nursing diagnoses associated with the individualized plan of care.
- EBP approaches in developing plans of care include the use of the Association of periOperative Registered Nurses (AORN) Guidelines for Perioperative Practice.
- Each guideline summarizes research and nonresearch evidence supporting best practices around a clinical question or topic guiding the selection of nursing interventions that lead to expected patient outcomes.

MEASURABLE PATIENT OUTCOMES

- In this section, standards of perioperative nursing, the use of standardized nursing language, surgical conscience, and fostering a culture of safety are discussed as each relates to the perioperative nurses' role in achieving measurable patient outcomes.
- The achievement of positive patient outcomes is central to nursing practice.

Standards of Perioperative Nursing

- According to AORN Guidelines for Perioperative Practice, the perioperative nurse should perform the following: Acquire specialized knowledge associated with the various types of surgical services; adhere to ethical principles and standards of practice; advocate for patients; collaborate with all members of the surgical team to promote positive patient outcomes; collect data and documents thoroughly in the legal health record; contribute to personal growth and the development of the self and peers; cultivate a healthy work environment; identify trends related to quality, patient safety, and provision of care; incorporate research into practice; provide leadership in the practice setting; systematically review the quality of care; use standardized nursing language in the documentation and planning of patient care; and utilize resources in a cost-efficient manner.
- The standards of perioperative nursing are focused on the provision of nursing care and the roles of the nurse. The standards apply to all nurses.
- The standards are developed by AORN and align with the American Nurses Association's (ANA's) scope and standards of practice.

Standardized Nursing Language

- The AORN developed the PNDS, a standardized nomenclature, to support perioperative nursing practice across the continuum. The nurse selects PNDS data elements and definitions as appropriate to influence patient outcomes.
- An example of an outcome statement using the PNDS: The patient will be free from signs and symptoms of surgical infection.

Surgical Conscience

- Surgical conscience requires the perioperative nurse to be engaged in continuous self-inspection coupled with the moral obligation to protect the patient.
- Surgical conscience consists of the following: adherence to standards from regulatory bodies; commitment to high values, sense of duty, and ethical practice; engaging in good personal hygiene and healthcare practices; engaging in the correction of errors as soon as they are known (i.e., breaks in technique); establishing a rapport with the patient and family members; maintaining accountability to the patient, employer, facility, profession of nursing, and the self; monitoring of one's own professional behavior as well as others on the surgical team; practicing in accordance with facility policy and standards of practice; promotion of patient advocacy and attending to the needs of the family; and shared responsibility to ensure that the principles of asepsis and sterile technique are observed.

Fostering a Culture of Safety

- A culture of safety is supported by the organization's leadership and encourages the following: acquiring appropriate resources and staff to safely complete the work; avoidance of placing blame; collaboration among all team members; eliminating workplace violence (i.e., bullying, incivility, and horizontal or lateral violence); promotion of transparency, accountability, and teamwork; trust among the members of the surgical team.

THE INDIVIDUALIZED PLAN OF CARE

- The individualized plan of care is created at the time of the preoperative interview and is based on the type of surgery to be performed, the positioning needed to optimize the exposure of the surgical site, and specific needs associated with safety promotion.
- The perioperative nurse should develop an individualized plan of care that incorporates the use of the following: assessment data from the preoperative interview; cultural sensitivity; NANDA guidance and diagnoses listing; Perioperative Patient Focused Model; PNDS; and the nursing process (assessment, nursing diagnosis, planning, intervention, and evaluation).
- The nurse creates the individualized plan of care based on the type of surgery. Many of these categories can include the use of robotics.
- *Cardiothoracic surgery:* Procedures that consist of repairs to the heart (e.g., coronary artery bypass graft).
- *Craniotomy:* Procedures that focus on surgical intervention involving the brain or cranial bones.
- *General and gynecology:* Typically focused on the organs of the abdomen and pelvis.
- *Endoscopy:* Procedures that use an endoscope and are focused on the alimentary canal.
- *Neurosurgery:* Procedures that are focused on the nerves.
- *Spinal surgery:* Procedures that focus on the repair of the vertebra and the spinal column.
- *Ophthalmic surgery:* Procedures that focus on the repair of issues associated with the eyes.
- *Organ procurement:* A procedure that is performed to procure organs for transplant and can consist of bone, eyes, and internal organs. Orthopedic surgery and sports medicine.
- *Otorhinolaryngologic surgery (head and neck):* Procedures that consist of repairs to structures in the head, ears, or throat. ▶

THE INDIVIDUALIZED PLAN OF CARE (*continued*)

- *Plastic and reconstructive surgery:* Procedures that consist of repairs to any part of the body (e.g., breast augmentation or removal, facial reconstruction).
- *Urologic surgery:* Procedures that consist of repairs to the kidneys, bladder, ureters, penis, prostate, tumor removal, including vaginal reconstruction and stent placement.
- *Vascular surgery:* Procedures performed to repair arteries or vasculature, or for stent or shunt placement.
- The patient's positioning needs, the draping required, and the instrumentation to be used are specific to the type of procedure to be performed.
- The type of anesthesia to be administered depends solely on the judgment of the anesthesia team in collaboration with the surgeon and the patient.

Assessment Data

- Assessment data consists of the information collected from the preoperative interview and focused physical assessment.
- Individualizing the plan of care requires creating measurable patient outcomes based on assessment data and nursing diagnoses.
- Identify measurable patient outcomes throughout the perioperative phases: preoperative, intraoperative, and postoperative. An example of an outcome statement for the individualized plan of care using the PNDS is, "The patient will remain free from thermal injury."
- The perioperative nurse should use patient assessment data and nursing diagnoses to guide the selection of appropriate nursing interventions, establish a baseline for measuring the interventions' achievement, select a time frame to measure the achievement of the goal, and collect data based on its relationship to the surgical intervention.

[UNFOLDING SCENARIO 3A]

Consider the following case study and the use of the nursing process.

A 20-year-old patient has been admitted directly to the presurgical holding area from the emergency department following a motor vehicle accident resulting in a head injury and a deep penetrating wound to the right leg. The patient is unconscious and unresponsive to noxious stimuli. The patient's mother confirms that the patient has no allergies or previous surgical history, is a nonsmoker, drinks on occasion, takes no medications, weighs 185 lb., and is 5 ft. 11 in. tall. The emergency department has removed all piercings. The surgeon states that the right leg will need to be amputated. Warm blankets are placed on the patient, and the patient is prepared for transport to the OR.

Question

What other aspects of the assessment are necessary?

Cultural Sensitivity

- The perioperative nurse should write culturally sensitive, age-appropriate, realistic, and measurable outcomes with interdisciplinary input, incorporating patient and family expectations. ▶

Cultural Sensitivity (continued)

■ Ensure the plan of care addresses patient-specific problems or considerations, including the following: age-specific considerations (children and older adult patients require specific considerations related to positioning and normothermia); behavioral and physiologic reactions; community or social program accessibility (the patient's motivation to be proactive in postsurgical rehabilitation is influenced by access to care); cultural, ethnic, and religious impact on care; disease process implications; family pattern concerns and patient and family coping skills including suspected abuse; gender identification and history associated with gender transition therapy or surgery; and ineffective family coping related to the surgical intervention, which can create preoperative anxiety for the patient and impact postoperative healing.

North American Nursing Diagnosis Association Guidance and Diagnoses

■ NANDA diagnoses were developed in 1982 and are used to guide nurses and strengthen awareness related to the promotion of patient safety, improved patient outcomes, and quality of care.

■ The four types of NANDA diagnoses and examples of each are presented in Table 3.1.

■ Some of the most common NANDA nursing diagnoses for the perioperative setting are as follows. Table 3.2 details expected outcomes and appropriate nursing interventions for some of these diagnoses: acute pain, anxiety, deficient knowledge, hyperthermia and hypothermia, ineffective airway clearance, ineffective coping, ineffective peripheral tissue perfusion, impaired gas exchange, impaired urinary elimination, readiness for enhanced comfort, risk for allergy reaction, risk for aspiration, risk for delayed surgical recovery, risk for electrolyte imbalance, risk for hypothermia, risk for imbalanced fluid volume, risk for impaired skin integrity, risk for infection, risk for injury, and risk for perioperative positioning injury.

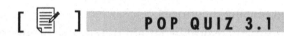

[▤]   **POP QUIZ 3.1**

Provide an example of a NANDA outcome statement related to electrical injury.

TABLE 3.1 NANDA Diagnoses		
NANDA DIAGNOSIS	**DESCRIPTION**	**EXAMPLE**
Health promotion	Goal to improve patient's overall health and well-being	Readiness for enhanced family coping related to surgical intervention
Problem-focused	Formulated during nursing assessment; chronic	Decreased cardiac output related to blood loss
Risk	Associated with development of a problem associated with the surgical intervention	Risk for imbalanced fluid volume related to blood loss
Syndrome	Associated with a pattern of issues related to the surgical intervention	Ineffective peripheral tissue perfusion related to blood loss

NANDA, North American Nursing Diagnosis Association.

TABLE 3.2 Common Nursing Diagnoses for the Perioperative Patient

NURSING DIAGNOSIS	EXPECTED OUTCOME	INTERVENTIONS
Anxiety	The patient will exhibit relaxed facial expressions and body movements.	• Address spiritual or cultural needs. • Assess anxiety level. • Explain the perioperative events. • Greet the patient and ask how they would like to be addressed. • Identify special concerns raised by the patient. • Offer emotional support and reassurance.
Risk for SSI	The patient will remain free from infection.	• Adhere to usage instructions for all perioperative skin prep. • Designate the appropriate wound classification. • Identify patient-specific risk factors associated with maintaining hemodynamic stability and skin integrity. • Maintain patient normothermia throughout the procedure. • Reduce traffic flow in the surgical suite. • Review the patient history and physical. • Use proper hand hygiene and aseptic technique. • Verify the sterility of all items introduced to the sterile field. • Verify that the room temperature is between 68°F and 75°F (20°C–23.9°C) and humidity is between 20% and 60%.
Risk for thermal injury	The patient will be free from thermal injury.	• Apply a grounding pad to protect the patient from electrical current. • Clean and dry skin prior to applying dressings. Remove all hair from the surgical site as indicated by the surgeon. • Preserve skin integrity. • Protect the patient from thermal, electrical, laser, and chemical injury in accordance with facility guidelines and manufacturer's instructions for equipment use. • Remove blood and body fluids from around the patient and apply a clean gown and blankets before transfer.
Risk for positioning injury	The patient will be free from signs and symptoms of positioning injury.	• Adjust the surgical table to meet the needs of the size of the patient. • Assess the patient for range of motion issues, prosthetics, and corrective devices. • Lift and transport the patient using the appropriate assistive equipment and personnel. • Reassess the patient for signs and symptoms of injury. • Use proper body alignment when positioning the patient and in consideration of limitations.

(*continued*)

TABLE 3.2 Common Nursing Diagnoses for the Perioperative Patient (*continued*)		
NURSING DIAGNOSIS	**EXPECTED OUTCOME**	**INTERVENTIONS**
Risk for imbalanced fluid volume	The patient will maintain normal fluid volume during the surgical procedure.	• Assist anesthesia personnel with the collection of laboratory samples as needed. • Collaborate with the surgeon and anesthesia team on fluid replacement therapies. • Communicate blood loss through sponge count and suction container contents. • Review orders for blood and blood products and have them available or easily accessible prior to the procedure.
Risk for impaired tissue integrity	The patient's skin will remain intact.	• Apply dressings according to the surgeon's preferences to clean and dry skin. Assess the surgical incision for bleeding, drainage, and tissue integrity along the suture line. • Assess the surgical site for color, redness, swelling, warmth, and the patient's report of pain. • Assess other areas of the body for signs of skin integrity issues associated with pressure, friction, and shear.
Risk for hypothermia	The patient will retain an intraoperative core temperature of 96°F–99°F (35.6°C–37.2°C).	• Adjust the room temperature and humidity to accommodate for the preservation of normal body temperature. • Collaborate with the surgical team and anesthesia team related to the use of warmed IV fluid and warm sterile fluid dispensed to the surgical field. • Use warm blankets and forced-air warming devices to maintain normothermia.

SSI, surgical site infection.

[UNFOLDING SCENARIO 3B]

The patient has been transferred to the OR suite where the surgical team awaits. Bleeding has been controlled, and the patient's vital signs (VS) are stable. Upon moving the patient to the OR table, the nurse notices that there is a profuse amount of blood coming through the dressing on the right leg.

Question

What nursing diagnoses would be considered for this patient?

Using the Perioperative Nursing Data Set for Outcome Identification

■ The National Library of Medicine defines PNDS as a "standardized nursing language [used] to support evidence-based perioperative nursing practice" (n.d., "Purpose").

■ PNDS is used to identify patient-specific diagnoses and select interventions for each to achieve expected outcomes including the following: nursing process framework, patient-specific disease processes, and patient-specific nursing diagnoses. ▶

Using the Perioperative Nursing Data Set for Outcome Identification (*continued*)

- PNDS has been integrated through AORN Syntegrity documentation to perform the following: Assist in the measurement and evaluation of patient outcomes, detect patient risks and associated evidence-based interventions, identify deficiencies in documentation, improve electronic documentation, standardize documentation by providing a universal language, support the creation of individualized patient-centered care plans, and support clinical practice.

Perioperative Patient-Focused Model

- The Perioperative Patient-Focused Model was developed by AORN and is an outcome-driven model used to describe the relationship between the perioperative nurse and the patient.

[ ]   **POP QUIZ 3.2**

What are the four main purposes of PNDS in perioperative documentation?

[UNFOLDING SCENARIO 3C]

The patient is rapidly prepped and draped. The results of the CT scan of the head indicate that the patient has a concussion, and no cranial bleed is present. The surgeon begins the surgical assessment of the right leg. The circulating nurse calls for the time-out, and the team participates by pausing and confirming the right patient, site, procedure, equipment, and needs for the case.

Question

What should the nurse plan for next related to this case?

- There are four domains in this model: Behavioral responses relate to the patient's behavioral response to perioperative care. Patient safety relates to the promotion of patient safety in the surgical environment. Physiologic responses relate to the patient's physiologic response to the surgical intervention. The health system relates to where the perioperative care is provided and the resources available.
- The model aligns with the standards of perioperative nursing and addresses the responsibilities of the perioperative nurses who are associated with the role; the responsibility of each nurse to ensure that the work environment is safe and that adequate resources are available to provide care; and the requirement for the nurse to provide individualized care that is designed to meet unique patient needs, prevent injury, and encompass sensitivity to culture, race, ethnic diversity, and patient preference.

The Nursing Process

- The perioperative nurse should document the ADPIE (common mnemonics are ADPIE and ANPIE), which stands for assessment, diagnosis, planning, implementation, and evaluation. Assessment includes a review of the medical record, validation of important findings, collaboration with the patient, and accurate

[ ]   **NURSING PEARL**

Patient outcome statements are derived from the nursing diagnoses and formulated by collaborating with the patient, family members, and other members of the healthcare team.

interpretation of clinical data. The nursing diagnosis requires the synthesis of the data collected and the formulation of a clinical judgment. Outcome identification in perioperative nursing is focused on preventative methods and generalized to all patients undergoing surgery. Planning is associated with the formulation of nursing interventions to address the needs of the patient during all phases of perioperative care. Evaluation is an ongoing process and incorporates the identification of outcomes that were met and those that will be communicated as needed to be met during handoff to the PACU. ▶

The Nursing Process (*continued*)

■ The documentation of patient care should include all aspects of the nursing process. The achievement of outcomes, as well as outcomes yet to be met, should be communicated to all members of the patient care team.

[ ]   **NURSING PEARL**

Ida Jean Orlando-Pelletier introduced the well-known and universally used five stages of the deliberative nursing process theory:

- Assessment
- Diagnosis
- Planning
- Implementation
- Evaluation

This process is sometimes called ADPIE.

[UNFOLDING SCENARIO 3D]

The amputation is complete, and the specimen is packaged for transport to pathology. The patient's VS remain stable, and no transfusion is needed. The surgeon and nurse first assistant begin primary closure of the wound. The scrub personnel begin to organize the instruments on the table.

Question

What is the nurse's next action?

[UNFOLDING SCENARIO 3E]

The surgical counts are completed and identified as correct. The dressings are applied, and a passive surgical drain is sutured into place by the surgeon. The nurse notices a pooling of prep solution under the thigh and blood on the gown.

Question

What is the nurse's next action?

RESOURCES

AORN Syntegrity. (2021). *Standardized nursing documentation with perioperative nursing data set (PNDS)*. https://www.aorn.org/syntegrity/products

Association of periOperative Registered Nurses. (2018). *PNDS (Perioperative nursing data set) – synopsis*. [Data set]. National Library of Medicine.

Association of periOperative Registered Nurses. (2019). *Guideline essentials: Key takeaways*. [Poster/implementation tool]. https://www.aorn.org/essentials/information-management

Association of periOperative Registered Nurses. (2021a). *2021 guidelines for perioperative practice*. Author.

Association of periOperative Registered Nurses. (2021b). *Environment of care (AORN guideline)*. https://aornguidelines.org/guidelines/content?sectionid=173720645&view=book#229132499

Nursing Theory. (n.d.). *Ida Jean Orlando – Nursing theorist*. https://nursing-theory.org/nursing-theorists/Ida-Jean-Orlando.php

Phillips, N., & Hornacky, A. (2021). *Berry and Kohn's operating room technique* (14th ed.). Elsevier.

Rothrock, J. C., & McEwen, D. R. (Eds.). (2019). *Alexander's care of the patient in surgery* (16th ed.). Elsevier.

4 INTRAOPERATIVE PATIENT CARE AND SAFETY

OVERVIEW

- There are many interventions and actions needed for the perioperative nurse to complete in the intraoperative phase. In this chapter, the following topics are reviewed: the time-out process, patient positioning, ergonomics and body mechanics, anesthesia management, surgical counts, surgical site management, management of equipment, management of implants and explants, and intraoperative blood transfusion and salvage.
- *Note:* Throughout each phase of the perioperative experience, the nurse will perform duties using the ACE process: Assess, Confirm, and Evaluate and Ensure.

NURSE'S ROLE IN PATIENT CARE AND SAFETY

- The perioperative nurse serves many roles related to providing patient care and ensuring safety. These roles include patient advocate, observer, circulator, scrub, and manager of the surgical suite.
- The goal of perioperative nursing is to provide patients with a level of care that is collaborative, uses the most current evidence-based practice guidelines, enhances safety, is competent and makes use of critical thinking, and is patient centered.

Assess

- Assessment of the perioperative patient is ongoing throughout the perioperative period and consists of the following: customizing care based on the patient's unique needs and the individualized needs of the procedure; promoting physiologic and psychologic homeostasis; providing privacy and dignity to the patient and their family members; and reducing stressful factors associated with the surgical environment.
- The primary function of the nurse related to continuous surgical field and intraoperative activity consists of the following: continuous assessment of the temperature and humidity in the surgical suite and reporting deviations from the facility and unit-based protocol; evaluating procedure product and equipment packaging to ensure sterility parameters have been met; limiting staff movement within or outside of the sterile field to prevent the breach of sterility; performing equipment function testing to ensure functionality; and reducing the risk of slip and fall and fire by performing an environmental scan.

Confirm

- Confirm that all patient safety needs have been addressed by the following: communicating to all levels of staff to ensure safety using standard handoff protocols; disseminating and verifying the receipt of patient information; developing and supporting a proactive approach to solving problems rather than a reactive and blaming approach; encouraging a sense of trust among all team members through effective communication and adherence to policy and procedure; and having a commitment to affirming and making patient safety a priority.

Evaluate and Ensure

- The role of the perioperative nurse in promoting safety and providing patient care involves continuous evaluation of the following: environmental health hazards on and off the field; equipment functionality; location and placement of sharps, sponges, and other items that have the potential to be retained within a cavity; patient's well-being during the continuum of care (e.g., blood loss, changes in vital signs (VS), need for hemostatic agents); and surgeon's needs and preferences for the case.
- The perioperative nurse also ensures that the following measures are taken to promote patient safety: ensuring that the time-out process is performed, and limiting the traffic and monitoring movement in the three areas of the surgical unit—unrestricted, semi-restricted, and restricted.

TIME-OUT PROCESS

- The time-out process is the second phase of the Universal Protocol and is a team approach used to promote patient safety by ensuring the correct procedure is being performed on the correct patient.
- The purpose of the time-out is to prevent harm to the patient related to operating on the wrong site, operating on the wrong patient, or performing the wrong procedure.
- The time-out should occur after the patient has been prepped and draped for surgery and just before the surgical incision.

 ALERT!

The time-out process is one of the three phases of the Universal Protocol. The other aspects of the Universal Protocol, occurring before the patient is transported to the surgical suite, are conducting a preprocedure verification process and marking the procedural site. As of 2004, The Joint Commission (TJC) identified that the Universal Protocol for Preventing Wrong Site, Wrong Procedure, Wrong Person Surgery is required for all accredited organizations.

Assess

[UNFOLDING SCENARIO 4A]

A 28-year-old patient has been transferred to the surgical suite for arthroscopic anterior cruciate ligament (ACL) repair on the right knee. The patient is intubated, and a right femoral block is performed. The patient is positioned in the hemi-lithotomy position according to the surgeon's preference and is prepped and draped for surgery. The surgeon states that she is ready to begin.

Question

What should the perioperative nurse do next?

- Assess the activity in the room and ensure that all members of the surgical team are ready to conduct the time-out.
- If a patient has refused site marking or if site marking is impractical due to the nature of the surgery, adhere to the facility's policies and procedures.
- Examples of situations where marking may not be possible are as follows: dental surgery; interventional procedures (e.g., cardiac catheterization, pacemaker insertion); surgery on infants, as the marking may leave a permanent stain on the skin; and surgery on mucosal surfaces, perineum, or internal organs (e.g., kidney, lung, ureter).

Confirm

- Confirm the following: designated person on the team begins the time-out process; identity of the patient, the name of the procedure, incision site, presence of consent, and the visibility of the site marking; involvement of all surgical team members; use of a time-out for surgical cases where more than one surgery will be performed and when more than one surgeon is performing surgery; and use of a standardized process.

Evaluate and Ensure

- Evaluate the activity in the room and ensure that the following activities occur: A fire and safety risk assessment has been performed and confirmed with the surgeon; all equipment needed for the procedure is available, and concerns have been verbalized; antibiotic prophylaxis has been administered within 1 hr of the initial surgical incision; relevant radiographic images are properly labeled and displayed where the team can see them; introduction of the surgical team members has been completed; surgical instrumentation to be used is confirmed as being sterile; the patient has been positioned to maximize the exposure of the surgical site; the surgeon has verbalized anticipated critical events (e.g., critical or nonroutine steps, a longer duration of the case, anticipated blood loss); the sterilization indicators are present, viable, and visible, thus indicating that sterilization parameters have been met.

[ ] **NURSING PEARL**

I PASS CARE Mnemonic for Time-Out
- Introduce the team
- Procedure
- Assessment for fire and safety
- Site confirmed and marked
- Sterilization
- Consent
- Antibiotics administered
- Radiographs displayed
- Equipment available

[UNFOLDING SCENARIO 4B]

During the time-out process, the surgeon requests the x-rays and MRI image results.

Question

What should the perioperative nurse do?

PATIENT POSITIONING

- Patient positioning is a collaborative process that involves all surgical team members. The process consists of the following: Thorough preoperative assessment, selection of the appropriate equipment, thorough postoperative evaluation of the patient after positioning is complete and before surgical draping, and documentation of the positioning process and materials used.
- The goals of appropriate patient positioning are to perform the following: Maintain the patient's privacy and comfort; maximize surgical site exposure; promote access to the intravenous (IV) lines for anesthesia and monitoring; stabilize the patient to prevent friction and shear to the skin and patient shift during surgery; maximize circulation and oxygenation; promote perfusion to all vital organs and extremities; and protect the muscles, nerves, skin, joints, and vital organs from injury.

Assess

- Assess for potential positioning injuries related to the following: Cold can reduce peripheral circulation, reduce oxygen delivery, and affect the skin and underlying tissue. Heat can increase tissue metabolism, increase oxygen demand, and constrict or impede blood flow. Moisture can macerate tissue, causing the connective tissue to dissolve and tear. Moisture can present as patient perspiration, irrigants, blood, urine, fecal matter, or skin prep solution.

- Assess surgical positioning for potential yet common positioning injuries, such as stretching or compression of the brachial plexus, peroneal, and facial nerves.

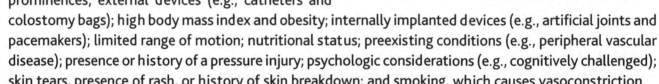

[🌐]   NURSING PEARL

The pressure-relieving surface associated with positioning devices disperses the patient's body weight, alleviates pressure on bony prominences, and reduces pressure on the areas that are touching the OR table.

- During the assessment, consider the risks for positioning injuries, such as those with bony prominences; external devices (e.g., catheters and colostomy bags); high body mass index and obesity; internally implanted devices (e.g., artificial joints and pacemakers); limited range of motion; nutritional status; preexisting conditions (e.g., peripheral vascular disease); presence or history of a pressure injury; psychologic considerations (e.g., cognitively challenged); skin tears, presence of rash, or history of skin breakdown; and smoking, which causes vasoconstriction.

- Assess and select positioning equipment: Select equipment based on surgeon preference list and special requests made by the surgeon, ensure all equipment and positioning aids are operational and intact and will not cause harm to the patient, and inspect and maintain equipment on a regular basis and remove it from use if found nonoperational or damaged.

Confirm

- Confirm the appropriate positioning equipment is available based on the planned surgical positioning (Table 4.1).

TABLE 4.1 Common Patient Positions for Surgery

POSITION	DESCRIPTION	POSITIONING EQUIPMENT	AREAS OF OPTIMAL ACCESS
Supine	• The patient is lying flat on the back on the surgical table in an anatomic position. • Special attention should be placed on the position of the arms/hands. ◦ Palm up for traditional supine with arms extended ◦ Palms facing torso if tucked to side *Note*: If the arms are to be tucked for the procedure, use a sled positioner or be sure that there is a long enough draw sheet.	• Bilateral arm boards (if required) • Foam or gel headrest • Gel pads • Foam or gel pad or blanket to elevate heels • Foam or gel knee positioner or blanket placed behind the knee to elevate the leg • Safety straps	• Abdomen ◦ Abdominoplasty ◦ Appendectomy ◦ Cholecystectomy ◦ Laparoscopic abdominal procedures • Head ◦ Craniotomy ◦ Sinus surgery

(continued)

TABLE 4.1 Common Patient Positions for Surgery (*continued*)			
POSITION	**DESCRIPTION**	**POSITIONING EQUIPMENT**	**AREAS OF OPTIMAL ACCESS**

Trendelenburg	• This is a commonly used position for abdominal surgeries that causes an elevation in cerebral blood and cerebrospinal fluid volume where the torso is lower than the legs.
	• The patient is lying on the back on the surgical table in an anatomic position.
	• The table is tilted with the head lower than the feet.
		• Bilateral arm boards (if required)
		• Foam or gel headrest
		• Gel pads
		• Foam or gel pad or blanket to elevate heels
		• Foam or gel knee positioner or blanket placed behind the knee to elevate the leg
		• Safety straps
			• Abdomen
			  ◦ Colorectal surgery
			  ◦ Gynecology procedures
			  ◦ Laparoscopic abdominal procedures
			• Pelvis
			  ◦ Robotic prostate surgery

Reverse Trendelenburg	• This is a position where the surgical site is elevated above the heart to improve drainage of fluids away from the site. This reduces intracranial pressure and improves pulmonary function where the torso is higher than the feet.
	• The patient is lying on the back on the surgical table in an anatomic position.
	• The table is tilted with the feet lower than the head.
		• Bilateral arm boards (if required)
		• Foam or gel headrest
		• Gel pads
		• Foam (or gel) pad or blanket to elevate heels
		• Foam or gel knee positioner or blanket placed behind the knee to elevate the leg
		• Padded footboard
		• Safety straps
			• Abdomen
			  ◦ Bariatric surgery
			  ◦ Laparoscopic abdominal procedures
			• Head and neck surgery

Sitting and modified sitting	• In this position, the patient is sitting with the head, neck, and torso elevated at 20° to 90°, the hips are flexed between 45° and 60°, and the knees flexed 30°.
	• The patient is in a sitting position. This position is also known as Fowler's, semi-Fowler's, high-Fowler's, and beach chair.
		• Foam or gel headrest or padding to protect the occiput, scapulae, and ischial tuberosities
		• Foam or gel pads
		• Knee positioner to protect the back of the knees
		• Foam or gel pad under the ankles to elevate the heels
		• Footboard with foam or gel padding to prevent sliding and protect the feet
		• Safety straps
			• Chest
			  ◦ Breast reduction
			• Head
			  ◦ Nasal surgeries
			• Shoulder
			  ◦ Shoulder arthroscopy and replacement

(*continued*)

TABLE 4.1 Common Patient Positions for Surgery (*continued*)

POSITION	DESCRIPTION	POSITIONING EQUIPMENT	AREAS OF OPTIMAL ACCESS

Lithotomy	• This position offers exposure to the vagina, rectum, and perineum through the use of stirrups for the legs. The upper body and torso are positioned flat on the surface of the OR table. There are five levels of lithotomy:
	• Low: The patient's hips are flexed and lower legs are parallel with the OR table.
	• Standard: The patient's hips are flexed at 80° to 100° and the lower legs are parallel with the OR table.
	• Hemi: The patient's nonoperative leg is positioned in a supine and flat position while the operative leg is in traction or another positioning device (i.e., fracture table).
	• High: The patient's hips are flexed and the stirrups are fully elevated.
	• Exaggerated: The patient's hips are flexed and the lower legs are almost at a vertical position.
		• Foam or gel headrest
		• Foam or gel pads
		• Bilateral arm boards (if required)
		• Padded stirrups to be positioned at the same height to avoid back strain and hip dislocation
		• Candy cane stirrups may also be used (although not a current standard of practice)
		  ○ The patient's legs should be padded where the leg rests on the metal of the stirrup.
		• Safety straps
			• Abdomen
			  ○ Colon surgery (low anterior colectomy)
			• Pelvis
			  ○ Gynecology procedures
			  ○ Childbirth
			  ○ Hysterectomy
			  ○ Removal of bladder
			  ○ Urology procedures

Prone	• This position provides exposure to the sacral, rectal, or perineal areas and is also used for spinal procedures due to the reduction in abdominal pressure it affords.
	• The patient is lying on the stomach.
		• Foam or gel headrest
		• Foam or gel pads
		• Foam or gel positioners, gel rolls, or blanket rolls (also known as chest rolls) under the shoulders, bilaterally
		• Foam or gel knee pads
		• Padded arm boards
		• Foam or gel positioner under the ankles to elevate the feet
		• Safety straps
			• Back
			  ○ Neurospine and cranial/brain surgery
			• Extremities
			  ○ Surgery on the posterior aspect of the extremities
			• Rectal surgery

(*continued*)

TABLE 4.1 Common Patient Positions for Surgery (*continued*)

POSITION	DESCRIPTION	POSITIONING EQUIPMENT	AREAS OF OPTIMAL ACCESS
Jackknife/Kraske	• The patient is lying on the stomach and the surgical table is lowered at the waist. The patient's head and feet are lower than the hips.	• Foam or gel headrest • Foam or gel pads • Foam or gel positioners or blanket rolls (also known as chest rolls) under the shoulders, bilaterally • Foam or gel knee pads • Padded arm boards • Foam or gel positioner under the ankles to elevate feet • Safety straps	• Pelvis • Rectal procedures

Lateral	• In this position, the patient is lying on the side. The dependent side, which is lying on the OR table, is the nonoperative side.	• Foam or gel headrest
		• Foam or gel pads
		• Foam or gel positioners under the arms
		• Axillary roll under the rib cage, posterior to the axilla
		• Upper arm on a padded arm board
		• Lower arm resting on a separate arm board
		• Pillow between the legs and padding for the ankles and feet
		• Safety straps
			• Abdomen
			  • Kidney surgery
			  • Liver surgery
			• Chest
			  • Lobectomy
			• Thorax
			  • Thoracotomy
			• Extremities
			  • Hip arthroplasty

Kidney	• The patient is lying on the side with the affected side up.
	• The kidney post is elevated once the patient has been positioned.
		• Foam or gel headrest
		• Foam or gel pads
		• Foam or gel positioners under the arms
		• Axillary roll under the rib cage, posterior to the axilla
		• Upper arm on a padded arm board
		• Lower arm resting on a separate arm board
			• Abdomen
			  • Kidney surgery
			  • Liver surgery
			• Chest
			  • Lobectomy
			• Thorax
			  • Thoracotomy

(*continued*)

TABLE 4.1 Common Patient Positions for Surgery (*continued*)

POSITION	DESCRIPTION	POSITIONING EQUIPMENT	AREAS OF OPTIMAL ACCESS
		• Pillow between the legs and padding for the ankles and feet • Safety straps	

Fracture table	• The patient is lying flat on the surgical table from the lower back to the occiput. The arm on the operative side may be elevated in a sling or be secured across the chest (surgeon specific). The other arm is placed on a padded arm board or tucked. The nonoperative leg is placed in a padded leg holder. The operative leg is positioned in the traction boot.	• Foam or gel headrest
		• Foam or gel pads
		• Padded arm board
		• Extra padding for protection for all areas touching the bed
		• Safety straps
			• Lower extremities
			  · Hip fracture
			  · Hip: Intramedullary rod insertion
			  · Anterior hip arthroplasty

Knee–chest	• The patient can be lying lateral or prone. Prone and knee–chest position require additional padding for the knees and feet on a knee board.	• Foam or gel headrest
		• Foam or gel pads
		• Foam or gel positioners or blanket rolls (also known as chest rolls) under the shoulders, bilaterally
		• Foam or gel knee pads
		• Padded arm boards
		• Safety straps
			• Rectum
			  · Hemorrhoidectomy
			  · Pilonidal cyst removal

Wilson Frame	• A variation of the prone position to maximize exposure for spinal surgery. The chest and pelvis are elevated slightly.	• Foam or gel headrest
		• Foam or gel positioners or blanket rolls (also known as chest rolls) under the shoulders, bilaterally
		• Foam or gel knee pads
		• Padded arm boards
		• Foam or gel positioner under the ankles to elevate the feet
		• Safety straps
			• Back
			  · Neurospine surgery
			• Extremities
			  · Surgery on the posterior aspect of the extremities
			  · Rectal surgery
			• Rectum
			  · Hemorrhoidectomy
			  · Pilonidal cyst removal

Evaluate and Ensure

- Evaluate the patient who is at higher risk for positioning complications, such as those who are obese. Obese patients are at higher risk for airway compromise, difficult intubation, aspiration, hypoxia, cardiac issues, skin breakdown, and intraabdominal pressure. Obese patients may require special equipment related to positioning, such as procedure beds that have a higher weight capacity, extra-long and wide safety straps, additional side-of-the-bed attachments, and additional positioning aids.

- Evaluate and ensure patients are protected from common positioning injuries, such as those that impact the cardiovascular system, eyes, internal organs, nerves, lungs, and skin.

- Evaluate and ensure that the patient is protected from changes in temperature, moisture, and pressure. Changes in temperature and heat exposure cause an increase in metabolism, which can impact blood loss. changes in anesthesia drug metabolism. and adverse cardiac events. Excessive exposure to cold room temperatures or solutions can cause hypothermia. Moisture can produce maceration of the skin and skin breakdown. Pressure from wrinkles in the sheets, extra padding and linens, and additional layers can injure the skin.

- Ensure the following occurs associated with protecting the patient from injury related to positioning: Apply appropriate head support for the patient and avoid the use of towels or blankets that provide no cushion to the occiput; assess the patient's pulses before and after positioning; avoid extreme lateral rotation of the patient's head; avoid contact between the patient and the metal aspects of the OR table; collaborate with anesthesia personnel to ensure protection of the patient's airway at all times; continuously monitor the position of the patient's hands and fingers during all phases of positioning; do not allow equipment or heavy objects to rest on the patient; do not lean on the patient; do not allow the patient's extremities to fall below the level of the or table; ensure that warming cabinet settings are consistent with the manufacturer's instructions for use (IFU) to prevent fire and thermal injury to the patient; and protect the patient's eyes with facility-approved eye protection or transparent dressings.

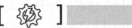

ALERT!

A thorough assessment of the patient after positioning should be completed to evaluate and ensure that all risks for injury have been addressed.

POP QUIZ 4.1

A 53-year-old female undergoes an elective total thyroidectomy for treatment of hypothyroidism. The patient is placed in the supine position with both arms tucked. What areas of the patient's body should the nurse pad to prevent injury?

[UNFOLDING SCENARIO 4C]

The patient undergoing a right knee arthroscopic ACL repair is to be placed in the hemi-lithotomy position according to the surgeon's preference. The patient weighs 125 lb. and is 5 ft. 3 in. tall.

Question

What areas of the body should be padded?

ERGONOMICS AND BODY MECHANICS

Perioperative nurses need to utilize effective ergonomics and body mechanics while working in the surgical unit. The work performed in the surgical unit places a great degree of stress and strain on the body. By ensuring that appropriate ergonomic tools are used, the nurse promotes safety in the work environment.

Assess

- Assess the following pertaining to the surgical procedure: access to transfer devices; assistive personnel needed to safely transfer the patient to and from the stretcher to the OR table; equipment to be moved for the procedure; height and weight of the patient; patient's range of motion and ability to move independently; patient's risk for fall; and surgical position to be used for the procedure and associated positioning equipment needs.
- Assess the high-risk tasks involved with performing the procedure, such as patient transfer and positioning, holding retraction, and movement of equipment.

Confirm

- Confirm the following related to the use of appropriate body mechanics: All staff are using ergonomic tools to move patients safely. Effective communication is used to evaluate and ensure safe patient movement and reduce the risk of injury to staff members.
- Confirm that risk-reduction strategies have been considered, such as the following: Conduct an ergonomic assessment of the suite and overall work environment; participate in risk-reduction and quality improvement activities; request assistance when lifting a heavy load or heavy equipment; and report ergonomic and work environment safety hazards to supervisors.

Evaluate and Ensure

- Evaluate the physical stressors associated with patient or equipment movement, such as the following: awkward and static postures, which are associated with holding the patient, are steady for prepping and draping; forceful exertion or overexertion, which is associated with the transfer of heavy equipment; lifting or carrying heavy patients or equipment and instrumentation; long work hours; prolonged standing; and repetitive motions.
- Evaluate that the fundamentals of patient transfer are observed by all staff members and include the following considerations: Can the patient transfer without assistance? How many staff members are needed? What is the starting position? What is the final position? What is the patient's weight? What devices are needed?
- Ensure the following actions are considered to reduce risks associated with excessive standing: Adjust the height of the OR table; alternate sitting and standing when possible; prop feet on a stool if the procedure requires standing for more than 2 hr; use antifatigue mats where feasible; wear supportive footwear that does not change the shape of the foot, is spacious enough inside to move toes, and is shock absorbent.
- Ensure the following steps are considered when performing patient transfers: Proper body alignment is maintained; provide support to the patient's extremities and airway; the number of personnel is adequate to safely transfer the patient; use assistive devices to facilitate patient transfer from one surface to another; work as a team to reduce the risk of injury to all personnel.

 ALERT!

According to the Association of periOperative Registered Nurses' (AORN's) 2021 guidelines for safe patient handling and movement, high-risk perioperative nursing tasks are patient transfers, repositioning of patients, lifting and holding extremities, standing, holding retractors, lifting and moving equipment, and sustaining awkward positions for extended periods of time.

[**UNFOLDING SCENARIO 4D**]

The surgery on the patient undergoing the right knee arthroscopic ACL repair has been completed, and it is time to move the patient back to the supine position.

Question

What considerations should the nurse make when repositioning the patient?

ASSISTING WITH ANESTHESIA MANAGEMENT

The perioperative nurse assists the anesthesia personnel from the point of induction to extubation.

Assess

- Assess the following associated with the planned procedure: length of surgery, patient age, and physiologic status of the patient.
- Assess the planned position for the procedure: postoperative recovery time, previous experience and history with anesthesia, surgery planned, and type of anesthesia to be administered.
- Assess the following stages of anesthesia during the procedure: Stage 1—analgesia or disorientation. Stage 2—excitement or delirium. Stage 3—surgical anesthesia. Stage 4—respiratory arrest.
- Assess the following phases of anesthesia: Induction—begins with the administration of anesthesia and lasts until the surgical incision. Maintenance—occurs after the surgical incision and lasts until near completion. Emergence—begins as the patient awakens.

Confirm

- Confirm the patient's American Society of Anesthesiology (ASA) score with the anesthesia provider: ASA I—normal and healthy patient. ASA II—patient with mild systemic disease (smoker, social drinker, pregnancy, controlled diabetes, hypertension, mild lung disease, obesity). ASA III—patient with severe systemic disease (diabetes mellitus [DM], hypertension, morbid obesity, chronic obstructive pulmonary disease [COPD]). ASA IV—patient with severe systemic disease that is a constant threat to life (myocardial infarction, cerebrovascular attack, trans-ischemic attack within 3 months). ASA V—moribund patient who is not expected to survive without the surgery or operation (ruptured abdominal aortic aneurysm, thoracic aneurysm, massive trauma, intracranial bleed, ischemic bowel). ASA VI—patient who has been declared brain-dead and whose organs are being donated.

Evaluate and Ensure

- Ensure that the perioperative nurse is working within the scope of practice outlined in their state's nurse practice acts when asked to assist the anesthesia provider.
- Evaluate and ensure that the perioperative nurse supports the patient at the bedside. ▶

[ ]   **ALERT!**

The perioperative nurse should work within the scope of practice and cannot fulfill the dual roles of the circulator and local/moderate sedation monitoring nurse.

Evaluate and Ensure (*continued*)

- Evaluate the needs of the anesthesia staff during general anesthesia, local anesthesia, regional anesthesia, and moderate sedation/analgesia. General anesthesia: The perioperative nurse provides ancillary assistance to, and works under the guidance of, the anesthesia team during induction and emergence. The perioperative nurse may be required to apply cricoid pressure during intubation and serves as a support for the patient. Local anesthesia: The perioperative nurse may be required to provide patient monitoring during the administration of local anesthesia through application of monitoring devices (blood pressure cuff, pulse oximetry, electrocardiogram), evaluation and documentation of vital signs, and positioning of the patient to ensure maximum exposure for surgery and comfort while in position. Moderate sedation/analgesia: The perioperative nurse may be required to administer medications and assess VS at prescribed intervals during the procedure. Regional anesthesia: The perioperative nurse may be required to assist during regional anesthesia through assessment of the type of medication used, assisting with the placement of monitoring devices, evaluation and assessment of vital signs, and supporting the patient during positioning (e.g., spinal placement).
- Evaluate the needs of the anesthesia personnel related to patient reactions and the risks associated with anesthesia such as bradycardia, fever, hematoma, hypotension, local anesthetic systemic toxicity, nausea and vomiting, postdural puncture headache, pruritus, shivering, and urinary retention.
- Ensure the following nursing interventions are provided during the course of the procedure: Ensure the safety of the environment; comfort the patient; set up equipment and obtain blood products, if needed; maintain the integrity of the sterile field; assist by initiating the flow of IV, if clamped off; facilitate intubation by holding for cricoid pressure (general anesthesia); assist with induction and emergence (general anesthesia or moderate sedation); assist with suction; and ensure safe handling and dispensation of medications and sharps during the course of the procedure and to the sterile field.

ALERT!

The perioperative nurse should review the plan for anesthesia with the anesthesia team and the surgeon related to the medications to be used, the route of administration, the length of the procedure, and other risk-related concerns.

NURSING PEARL

Surgical patients have significant anxiety when entering the surgical suite; therefore, the perioperative nurse plays an important role in reducing this anxiety and assisting the anesthesia staff to deliver safe effective care.

SURGICAL COUNTS

- The unintended retention of foreign objects remains the top-reported sentinel event through TJC.
- Ensuring counts of surgical items at risk for retention based on the procedure are completed reduces the risk of foreign object retention in the patient.

ALERT!

There may be exceptions to instrument counting per facility policy.

Assess

Assess the surgical field and perform the surgical count as follows (based on the surgical procedure):

- Before the start of the surgical procedure
- Upon dispensing sharps, sponges, or instrumentation to the surgical field
- Upon closing a cavity within a cavity
- Upon closing the first layer (e.g., fascia)
- Upon final closure
- When permanent relief of either a scrub person or nurse circulator occurs

Confirm

- Confirm the count between the scrub person and nurse circulator. If a counting error exists, identify errors in counting immediately and report them to the surgeon, stop all activity and begin a recount, and follow facility policy associated with counts that cannot be reconciled.
- Confirm that the instruments and devices are intact when they are returned to the field from the operative site.
- Verify the integrity and completeness of all items when counting.

Evaluate and Ensure

- Evaluate the surgical site and remove all soft goods, instruments, and sharps before counting. Key items to remember are as follows: Do not use towels inside the wound. Sponges should be radiopaque. When the wound is intentionally packed with radiopaque or nonradiopaque sponges, document the count once confirmed with the surgeon and communicate the number of retained sponges to the receiving unit.

[ ]   **ALERT!**

Both the circulator and scrub must be able to visualize all items during the count. Do not count product packages. The nurse circulator and the scrub person must count all physical soft goods, sharps, and instruments.

- Ensure that counts are not being performed during critical times during a procedure. *Note:* Anyone can call for an additional count at any time during the procedure. The surgeon has the authority to override the decision to perform a count during critical times. Adherence to hospital policy must be maintained.
- Ensure that the circulating nurse can visibly see all items during the count.

STERILE FIELD MANAGEMENT

The principles of aseptic technique are associated with using all items that have been appropriately sterilized, stored in sterile areas, and only come into contact with persons who are authorized to handle sterile items.

Assess

Assess the following associated with maintaining sterility:

- All items for use in the procedure must be sterile.
- Assess the integrity of all items dispensed to the surgical field.
- Compromised barriers are considered contaminated.
- Draped tables are sterile only at the table level or top surface.
- Edges of a sterile wrapper or container are considered unsterile.

Confirm

- Confirm that only persons considered sterile are touching the sterile field. Gowns have established parameters of sterility: Restrict movement around the sterile field.
- Confirm that the donning of gloves and gowns adheres to AORN recommendations and facility policy, hand hygiene is performed, inspection of the integrity of the gown and gloves has been performed, removal of contaminated gloves or gown is done promptly, selection of the surgical gown is associated with the degree of exposure, and sterile technique is followed when donning the gown and gloves.

Evaluate and Ensure

- Evaluate the movement of all personnel in and around the sterile field.
- Evaluate the following associated with the preparation of the sterile field: Do not move the sterile field beyond the surgical suite where it was originally opened. Prepare the sterile field as close to the time of actual use as possible. Only sterile items should come into contact with the sterile field. Use an isolation technique when working in a procedure involving the bowel, resection of metastatic tumors, or infected tissue.
- Ensure the following protocol is maintained throughout the procedure: Limit traffic in the surgical suite and keep the OR suite doors shut. Limit exposure of the other materials in the sterile field when hydrotherapy or debridement with irrigation is occurring. Monitor for breaks in sterility. Open and deliver sterile items in a manner that serves to maintain sterility. Open the sterile items according to the manufacturer's IFU. Review and follow the facility's policy if case is delayed and follow the procedure for covering the field or portions of the field when not in use. Sterile persons must pass each other face-to-face or back-to-back and keep their lower arms up above the waist. Unsterile persons should not walk between areas of sterility.
- Ensure the scrubbed members of the surgical team do the following throughout the procedure: Avoid changing levels of the hands, table height, or OR table height; avoid turning the back on the sterile field; avoid folding of the arms, as no part of the hands or arms should be under the axilla; remain close to the sterile field; keep hands and arms above waist level; and use shielding devices when radiologic exposure is expected.

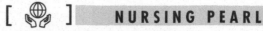

NURSING PEARL

When in doubt, throw it out! Any member of the surgical team can determine that there is a contamination. The more eyes on the sterile field and around the sterile field, the better. If there is uncertainty about any item, the intraoperative nurse should discard the disposable item or return the instrumentation to sterile processing in accordance with facility policy and procedure.

POP QUIZ 4.2

The scrub nurse performs a check of sharps during a carotid endarterectomy. The scrub alerts the circulating nurse and the surgeon that one of the vascular needles is missing. The surgeon states that this is a critical point in the procedure, and he cannot stop to do a full count. What is the circulating and scrub nurse's next action?

SURGICAL SITE MANAGEMENT

The perioperative nurse must work to reduce the risk of surgical site exposure to infectious materials.

Assess

- The circulating nurse and scrub person must continually assess the surgical site and area surrounding it to ensure that foreign bodies are not lost within a cavity or wound.
- Assessment activities include assessing the integrity of gloves and gowns worn by those at the surgical field, confining and containing spills to protect the integrity of the field and the tables, continuous evaluation of the integrity of surgical drapes, and monitoring for breaks in technique.

Confirm

Confirm all actions within the sterile field adhere to aseptic technique and work to maintain the sterility of the field, such as the following:

- Only scrubbed personnel should move within the sterile field.
- Sterile draping should cover all areas designated as the sterile field. ▶

Confirm (*continued*)

- Items used within the sterile field should be inspected first (expiration dates, sterilization indicators), then presented to the sterile field.
- Delivery of all items to the sterile field, including medications, should be performed using an aseptic technique.
- Traffic around the sterile field and within the surgical suite should be limited.

Evaluate and Ensure

- Evaluate the integrity of the following: gowns and drapes, sterile supply packaging, sterilization through the presence of external and internal sterilization indicators, and rigid container seals and locks.
- Ensure that the surgical wound is kept clean and free from packages, nonradiopaque sponges, and items not immediately used for the particular phase of surgery.

ALERT!

Foreign bodies left inside a patient's wound create serious harm. The surgical team should ensure that proactive risk strategies are used to prevent the occurrence of retained surgical items and work to reduce the risk for infection at the surgical site by maintaining the sterility of the field.

ALERT!

Effective in July 2019, these guidelines for surgical attire were approved by the AORN Guidelines Advisory Board.

PERSONAL PROTECTIVE EQUIPMENT

The personal protective equipment (PPE) and surgical attire worn in the OR should ensure a high level of cleanliness and hygiene, reduce the patient's exposure to microorganisms, reduce the risk for surgical site infection (SSI), and protect staff from cross contamination.

Assess

- Assess the integrity of surgical scrubs and ensure that only those that are laundered through the healthcare facility's approved site are used.
- Assess that all members of staff at the surgical field wear appropriate PPE such as eyewear, masks, and clean gowns.
- Ensure that gowns that are penetrated with blood or have experienced strikethrough from sharps are removed.

Confirm

- Confirm that the scrub attire is clean, covering areas of the body that shed (hair, arms, beard), nonlinting, safe for use (foot protection and shoes should adhere to Occupational Safety and Health Administration [OSHA] regulations and American Society for Testing and Materials [ASTM] F2414 standards), and stored in enclosed carts or containers and in a manner that prevents contamination.
- Confirm that PPE is fluid resistant (surgical gowns, gloves, and cover apparel), cleaned between cases if not disposable (specialty eye protection), and discarded after the case if disposable.

Evaluate and Ensure

- Evaluate the field for strikethrough and torn gloves.
- Ensure that breaks to the integrity of PPE are addressed promptly.
- Ensure staff is protected from cross contamination.

POP QUIZ 4.3

The scrub person is setting up the sterile field for an abdominal aortic aneurism procedure. As the circulating nurse requests to begin the surgical count, she notices that there is strikethrough on the scrub person's gown. What is the circulating nurse's next action?

ENVIRONMENTAL MANAGEMENT IN THE SURGICAL SUITE

Environmental management in the surgical suite includes the following:

- Chemical management (methyl methacrylate, glutaraldehyde, formaldehyde, formalin)
- Environmental cleaning
- Fire prevention
- Noise control and reduction
- Surgical smoke
- Thermal injury reduction

[ ]   **NURSING PEARL**

The fire triangle consists of the ignition source, the oxidizer, and the fuel source.

Assess

Assessment of the surgical environment is continuous and should address the following key areas related to the environment of care:

- Chemical management on and off the field
- Fire prevention and protection of patient from injury
- Level of noise occurring within the surgical suite
- Environmental cleaning to reduce the risk of infection
- Thermal injury reduction to the patient and staff

Confirm

Confirm the following are addressed:

[ ]   **ALERT!**

Surgical fires can occur at any location in the fire triangle. The perioperative nurse must know how to extinguish a fire and evacuate the OR and surgical suite.

- Chemical management on and off the field: A material safety data sheet (MSDS) should be available for all chemicals. Appropriate PPE (masks, gloves, and eyewear) should be worn when handling chemicals. Chemicals are stored in an area that is well ventilated and according to federal, state, and local regulations.
- Environmental cleaning: Cleaning should occur between each surgical case. Do not use spray bottles or brooms, as contamination can be spread through these methods. Environmental service personnel should follow surgical attire guidelines. Floors should be mopped with damp or wet mops. Selection of products should be done using a chemical hazard assessment. Terminal cleaning should occur at the end of the day. Use designated cleaning equipment.
- Fire prevention: Assess the type of skin prep used (is it flammable?). Assess types of ignition and fuel sources present (anesthesia gases, gases used in surgery, fluids used in surgery, electrocautery, drapes, gowns, the patient). Check testing of lasers or fiberoptic lighting and the spatial relationship to the drapes. Check the potential for the presence of high oxygen levels. Ensure that instruments and equipment to be used (electrocautery, heated probes, defibrillators, drills, saws, burrs) are not lying on the drapes.
- Noise control and reduction: Control the tone of conversations and extraneous distracting noise. Limit conversations that are not essential to the case. Limit the traffic within the surgical suite and the number of times the door is opened. Limit the use of communication devices, phones, and wireless systems. Reduce extraneous noise from music and equipment where feasible.
- Surgical smoke management: Evacuation of surgical smoke is performed by the surgical team. The smoke evacuation system is functioning and has a clean filter in place. PPE is worn when disposing of the filter. Wall suction should be operational and verified at the surgical field.
- Thermal injury reduction: Control the temperature of fluids used in the procedure. Implement a maximum temperature limit for blanket warming cabinets based on manufacturer guidelines. Monitor the placement of electrocautery instrumentation, fiberoptic cables, and laser equipment at the sterile field.

Evaluate and Ensure

- Evaluate that all safety measures are followed pertaining to facility policies and procedures.
- Ensure the following related to surgical skin prep and fire safety: Allow flammable skin antiseptics to dry completely and fumes to dissipate before surgical drapes are applied and before using a potential ignition source (e.g., electrical surgical unit [ESU], laser). Allow flammable solutions (e.g., alcohol, collodion, tinctures) to dry completely and fumes to dissipate before using an ignition source. Conduct a skin prep time-out to validate that the skin antiseptic is dry before draping the patient. Conduct, document, and communicate the completion of the fire risk assessment. Remove materials that are saturated with the skin antiseptic agent before draping the patient. Use reusable or disposable sterile towels to absorb drips and excess solution during application. Wick excess solution with a sterile towel to help dry the surgical prep area completely.

POP QUIZ 4.4

A 42-year-old female underwent a radical hysterectomy and sentinel node biopsy. The surgeon accidentally activates the monopolar current that was lying on the drape instead of the bipolar forceps. The foot pedals are pushed under the surgical table. A spark ignites the drape. What is the circulating nurse's first course of action?

MANAGEMENT OF EQUIPMENT AND MATERIALS

The perioperative nurse and surgical staff should use all equipment and surgical materials according to the manufacturer's recommendations.

Assess

Assess the function of all equipment to be used in a surgical case on and off the field.

Confirm

- Confirm that the special equipment to be used is available and functional.
- Confirm that required equipment has been tested preoperatively as appropriate.

Evaluate and Ensure

- Evaluate equipment, ensure its function, and examine for fire hazards: electrosurgery, lasers, pneumatic tourniquets, and ultrasonic instruments.
- Ensure that the surgical suite is made ready for the patient by the following processes: checking that the suite has IV poles and related equipment; collecting all intraoperative medications and dispensing them to the field using aseptic technique; dispensing supplies to the sterile field aseptically; leveling the surgical table and gathering all positioning equipment; selecting and examining sterile supplies according to the physician preference list; and testing the suction and making sure suction equipment is available.

ALERT!

Laser Safety

- The laser must display a warning label, per federal regulation.
- The laser aperture through which the laser beam is emitted must be clearly marked.
- When a laser filter is used in the microscope, the filter placement must be checked by two people, at least one of whom is a RN.
- The laser operator will be knowledgeable of and accountable for all laser safety in accordance with manufacturer instructions and facility policy and procedure.

MANAGEMENT OF IMPLANTS AND EXPLANTS

- Implants and explants should be handled using aseptic technique.
- Some devices require tracking. Facility policy and procedure manuals should outline the process of tracking, reporting, handling, returning, submitting to pathology, documenting, and disposing, as well as protocols on returning to patients.

Assess

- Assess the packaging of all implantable material before dispensing it to the surgical field.
- Assess the requirements for handling of explants related to final disposition.

Confirm

- Confirm with the surgeon the implant to be dispensed to the field. Autologous tissue management consists of the following: Facilities may be registered with the U.S. FDA as a tissue establishment, commonly referred to as a tissue bank. Facilities registered as tissue establishments must meet the laws outlined in the Code of Federal Regulations Chapter 21, Part 1271. In some states, tissue banks must be also licensed in that particular state and registered with the American Association of Tissue Banks (AATB).
- Confirm the explant identification with the surgeon.

Evaluate and Ensure

- Evaluate the special handling protocols of the implant according to the manufacturer's recommendations.
- Ensure that the information on the implant has been recorded for tissue tracking purposes, if applicable.
- Evaluate the following related to the handling of explants: chain of custody (e.g., forensic evidence), device failure and return to the manufacturer, and tissue tracking.

 ALERT!

There are times when law enforcement is waiting for evidence (e.g., knife fragments, bullet fragments). Adhere to facility policy and requirements of the law enforcement agency when handling these items.

INTRAOPERATIVE BLOOD TRANSFUSION AND SALVAGE

The intraoperative nurse should assess the need for blood salvage and blood products related to the surgical procedure.

Assess

- Assess for adverse effects associated with surgical bleeding, such as blood loss requiring blood transfusion, reduction in core body temperature, hypovolemic shock, thrombocytopenia, and visual obstruction at the surgical field.
- Assess the patient for the following issues associated with the use of hemostatic agents: allergies to any topical hemostatic agent or products of bovine or porcine origin; personal or family history of bleeding disorders, bleeding gums, easy bruising, excessive superficial bleeding, severe nosebleeds, anemia, or renal or hepatic disease; use of anticoagulants or anti-platelet (PLT) medications; use of aspirin-containing or other nonsteroidal anti-inflammatory prescription or over-the-counter medication; and use of supplements or herbs that might contribute to increased bleeding times.
- Assess the need for blood products using the TAPE mnemonic: **T**ype of procedure, **A**nticipated blood loss, **P**resence of type and cross match in the patient's lab results, and **E**valuation provided by the surgeon.

Confirm

- Confirm the patient's medication history related to the use of anticoagulants.
- Confirm the need for blood products with anesthesia personnel and the surgeon.

Evaluate and Ensure

- Evaluate the need for blood products and blood salvage. The objectives of transfusion are to increase circulating blood volume after surgery, trauma, or hemorrhage; increase the number of circulating red blood cells (RBCs) and maintain hemoglobin (HgB) levels in patients with anemia; and provide selected cellular components as replacement therapy.
- Evaluate the patient factors and procedural factors that contribute to surgical bleeding.
- Ensure that the requirements for blood transfusion are met: blood checked by two RNs or per institution policy, patient consent obtained, large gauge IV (#20 smallest) availability, patient response to transfusion (e.g., transfusion reactions and fluid volume excess), physician's order, VS to be taken as per institution policy, and secondary IV line with normal saline (NS) only.
- Ensure that assistance is provided to the surgeon to promote safe surgical hemostasis and reduce the risk for the need for infusion through the use of mechanical methods, pharmacologic agents, thermal- and energy-based methods, and topical hemostatic agents.

[]   **ALERT!**

- Transfusion reactions can happen immediately. Be vigilant in assessing the patient's VS posttransfusion.
- The use of hemostatic agents (topical and pharmacologic) is contraindicated for use during cell salvage.

SPECIMEN MANAGEMENT

- A specimen is any blood, soft tissue, bone, body fluid, or foreign body that has been ordered by the surgeon to be sent to the pathology lab for analysis.
- AORN recommends that the transfer of all specimens from the sterile field occur as soon as possible using sterile technique and standard precautions.
- AORN recommends that the integrity of the specimen is preserved during transfer.

Assess

- Assessment of specimen collection and special handling needs should begin when the procedure is scheduled.
- Assess that the process of specimen collection aligns with facility policy and incorporates a dedicated specimen collection process and transfer system, reduction in the number of people involved in the process, and standardized process.

Confirm

Confirm the following are completed related to specimen management:

- Breast cancer specimen handling should be streamlined and include the following related to documentation and disposition: time of excision and fixation (if required); transfer to pathology as soon as possible and record the time of transfer; and use of radiologic imaging (if needed).

[]   **ALERT!**

Specimen Containment Guidelines

- If one specimen container is compromised, it must be placed in a second leak-proof container.
- If the exterior surface of a container is considered contaminated during handling, it should be placed into a specimen bag.

Confirm (*continued*)

- Collection and handling of a specimen should be maintained in a manner that prevents misidentification or mishandling. Documentation and labeling should include the type of specimen and patient information (name, age, history, diagnosis); study required, date and time of collection, and information pertinent to the specimen; and surgeon's name and responsible party's signature.
- Patient and specimen identification should be made just before the removal of the specimen from the surgical field.
- Specimen containers should be labeled to communicate patient, specimen, preservative, and biohazard information.
- Tissue specimens should be designated for a routine pathologic examination, gross identification only, or disposal according to healthcare organization policies.

Evaluate and Ensure

- Evaluate the specimens and ask the surgeon how the specimen is to be handled (fixed or not fixed with a preservative).
- Evaluate special handling of forensic evidence.
- For highly infectious material, reduce the risk of exposure by alerting all healthcare professionals who might come in contact with the material (e.g., laboratory personnel other surgical team members); remove gloves and sanitize hands following the transfer of the specimen; and use standard precautions and PPE when handling all material.
- For Mohs procedure specimens, ensure that high-quality photographs are taken using a ruler, anatomic landmarks, and varied views under the guidance of the surgeon.
- Patients may request to retrieve placental tissue associated with live birth and related to cultural practices. Handle the specimen according to facility policy and ensure that it is refrigerated until it can be transferred to the pathology laboratory.
- For prion disease specimens, notify the pathology laboratory, sterile processing, and all surgical personnel who will be involved with the case when a patient with prion disease (e.g., Creutzfeldt-Jakob disease [CJD]) is scheduled. Perform in-person specimen handovers to pathology personnel, and use standard precautions and PPE when handling all materials associated with the case.
- For radioactive specimens, contain the specimen to prevent cross contamination, minimize the amount of handling involved, perform prompt transport of the specimen to the pathology laboratory and in accordance with facility policy, and record the presence of radioactive material on pathology requisition documentation.
- For umbilical cord blood, follow the facility policy for banked umbilical cord blood. Verify the disposition of umbilical cord blood and whether it is to be banked.
- Handling of specimens in formalin should follow facility policy and OSHA guidelines. *Formalin* is a clear solution of formaldehyde in water. A 37% solution is used for fixing and preserving biologic specimens for pathologic and histologic examination. Most specimens should be covered in formalin; however, some should not. Logging of the specimen should be completed according to facility policy, cultures should be handled appropriately, and specimens (tissue, fluid, bone, hardware) should be immediately passed off the field and placed in a labeled specimen container.

 ALERT!

AORN identified ALARA as a mnemonic to be used when handling radioactive specimens. ALARA = **A**s **L**ow **A**s **R**easonably **A**chievable.

 POP QUIZ 4.5

A 78-year-old male patient has been transferred to the OR for a right colectomy and lymph node excision. Near the end of the procedure, the scrub person notifies the circulating nurse that the specimens are ready for the handoff. The surgeon uses a suture to identify specific margins associated with the tumor removed in the colon. The scrub nurse hands off the colon specimen and the excised tumor in one bowl. The circulating nurse notices the markings on the tumor. What should the nurse do?

RESOURCES

21 CFR 1271. (2017). *Human cells, tissues, and cellular and tissue-based products*. Government Publishing Office.

Apple, B., & Letvak, S. (2021). Ergonomic challenges in the perioperative setting. *AORN Journal, 113*(4), 339–348. http://doi.org/10.1002/aorn.13345

Association of periOperative Registered Nurses. (2013a). *Recommended practices for maintaining a sterile field, perioperative standards and recommended practices*. Author.

Association of periOperative Registered Nurses. (2013b). *Recommended practices for prevention of retained surgical items, perioperative standards and recommended practices*. Author.

Association of periOperative Registered Nurses. (2019a). *AORN correct site surgery tool kit*. https://www.aorn.org/guidelines/clinical-resources/tool-kits/correct-site-surgery-tool-kit

Association of periOperative Registered Nurses. (2019b). *Guideline essentials: Key takeaways*. https://www.aorn.org/essentials/team-communication

Association of periOperative Registered Nurses. (2020). *Guideline for surgical attire, guidelines for perioperative practice*. Author.

Association of periOperative Registered Nurses. (2021a). *Guideline for a safe environment of care, guidelines for perioperative practice*. Author.

Association of periOperative Registered Nurses. (2021b). *Guideline for autologous tissue management, guidelines for perioperative practice*. Author.

Association of periOperative Registered Nurses. (2021c). *Position statement: Preventing wrong-patient, wrong-site, wrong-procedure events [Toolkit]*. https://www.aorn.org/-/media/aorn/guidelines/position-statements/posstat-wrong-site-0302.pdf

Association of periOperative Registered Nurses. (2021d). *Specimen management, guidelines for perioperative practice*. Author.

Hauk, L. (2018). Guideline for safe patient handling and movement. *AORN Journal, 107*, P10–P12. https://doi.org/10.1002/aorn.12287

Hughes, N. L., Nelson, A., Matz, M. A., & Lloyd, J. (2011). Safe patient handling and movement series. AORN ergonomic tool 4: Solutions for prolonged standing in perioperative settings. *AORN Journal, 93*(6), 767–774. https://doi.org/10.1016/j.aorn.2010.08.029

The Joint Commission. (n.d.). *The Universal Protocol*. https://www.jointcommission.org/standards/universal-protocol

The Joint Commission. (2021). *Summary data of sentinel events reviewed by The Joint Commission*. https://www.jointcommission.org/-/media/tjc/documents/resources/patient-safety-topics/sentinel-event/summary-se-report-2020.pdf

Rothrock, J. C. (2018). *Alexander's care of the patient in surgery* (16th ed.). Elsevier - Health Sciences Division.

Sona, C. (2013). Care of the surgical patient. In P. A. Potter & A. G. Perry (Eds.), *Fundamentals in nursing* (8th ed., pp. 1254–1294). Elsevier/Mosby.

Spera, P., Lloyd, J. D., Hernandez, E., Hughes, N., Peterson, C., Nelson, A., & Spratt, D. G. (2011). AORN ergonomic tool 5: Tissue retraction in the perioperative setting. *AORN Journal, 94*(1), 54–58. https://doi.org/10.1016/j.aorn.2010.08.031

Waters, T., Short, M., Llyod, J., Baptiste, A., Butler, L., Petersen, C., & Nelson, A. (2011). AORN ergonomic tool 2: Positioning and repositioning the supine patient on the OR bed. *AORN Journal, 93*(4), 445–449. https://doi/10.1016/j.aorn.2010.08.027

Waters, T., Spera, P., Peterson, C., Nelson, A., Hernandez, E., & Applegarth, S. (2011a). AORN ergonomic tool 3: Lifting and holding the patient's legs, arms, and head while prepping. *AORN Journal, 93*(5), 589–592. https://doi.org/10.1016/j.aorn.2010.08.028

Waters, T., Spera, P., Peterson, C., Nelson, A., Hernandez, E., & Applegarth, S. (2011b). AORN ergonomic tool 7: Pushing, pulling, and moving equipment on wheels. *AORN Journal, 94*(3), 254–260. https://doi.org/10.1016/j.aorn.2010.09.035

5 INTRAOPERATIVE PERSONNEL AND SERVICES

OVERVIEW

- There are many people involved in a surgical case. The role of the perioperative nurse is associated with the management of the case's personnel and services.
- This chapter focuses on the function of the interdisciplinary team and the role that the nurse plays in managing personnel and visitors.
- This chapter also includes a discussion of conflict management and the promotion of effective team collaboration and communication.
- Throughout each phase of the perioperative experience, the nurse will perform duties using the ACE process: Assess, Confirm, and Evaluate and Ensure.

FUNCTION OF THE INTERDISCIPLINARY TEAM

The interdisciplinary team functions to promote patient care, safety in the environment, and positive patient outcomes. An interdisciplinary surgical team may consist of, but is not limited to, the following personnel:

- Anesthesia personnel: anesthesiologist, certified registered nurse anesthetist (CRNA).
- Biomedical technicians: Their function is to provide support through maintenance of equipment and routine surveillance and testing of all mechanical equipment.
- Blood salvage technician: Their function is to operate the cell salvage equipment, maintain the equipment in conjunction with biomedical services, and report blood collection and critical issues to the surgeon and anesthesia personnel.
- Endoscopy technicians: Their function is to provide support to the physician of record (gastroenterologist) or surgeon during the case and maintain endoscopic equipment and camera sources.
- Materials management personnel: Their function is to stock sterile materials, place orders for materials used in surgery to achieve preset par levels, and communicate to the OR manager and appropriate team members.
- Sterile core technician or nurse: Their function is to maintain sterile stock orders, assemble case carts with supplies for scheduled cases, order special equipment as needed, and work with materials management personnel when there are delays in receiving materials needed for surgical cases per facility policy and procedure.
- Surgical assistants: These roles include medical assistant, registered nurse first assistant (RNFA), physician assistant (PA), APRN, nurse practitioner (NP), or surgical resident. Their function is to support the surgeon during the procedure and may perform surgical incision closure, depending upon the scope of practice for the state where the individual is practicing.
- Non-OR personnel: These roles include healthcare industry representative (HCIR), student observers, and medical residents. Their function consists of no formal role or function. HCIRs may offer guidance and instruction on the use of medical equipment and instrumentation. However, they are not permitted to touch any equipment, patient, or open any materials used in a procedure. ▶

FUNCTION OF THE INTERDISCIPLINARY TEAM (*continued*)

- Nursing roles include preoperative or intraoperative nurse (facility dependent), circulating nurse, scrub nurse, and RNFA.
- Nursing assistive personnel include anesthesia technicians and nursing assistive and OR technicians. Other emerging roles include surgical liaison, robotics coordinator, and nurse informaticist.
- Perfusionist: Their function is to operate extracorporeal circulation equipment (heart–lung machine) during open-heart surgery or any other procedure where artificial cardiac support is needed.
- Sterile processing technicians (also known as central service technicians): Their function is to prevent infection through sterilization, cleaning, processing, assembling, storing, and distributing the supplies to be used in surgery.
- Surgeon: Their function is to evaluate, diagnose, and treat conditions through surgical intervention.
- Surgical technologists (also known as OR technicians): Their function is to assist the surgeon by providing instrumentation, sharps, equipment, and other sterile materials.

Assess

- Assess the scope and practice function of each licensed and nonlicensed member of the surgical team.
- Assess the communication and collaboration efforts of the surgical team.

Confirm

- Confirm that the appropriate staffing is present in the surgical suite before transfer of the patient from preoperative holding, emergency department, or critical care unit.
- Confirm that the staffing for a surgical procedure is case dependent and may vary. Standard staffing for a surgical case is as follows: Anesthesia provider (during induction), circulating nurse, RNFA, scrub technician or nurse, and surgeon.
- Confirm that the appropriate staffing is present for handoff before and after the surgical case. Staffing is as follows, according to the surgical phase: For the preoperative phase, at least one RN. For the intraoperative phase, one RN (circulating nurse) and one scrub person (who may be an RN or surgical technologist). For postoperative phase I, two licensed nurses, possibly an RN and RN anesthetist. For postoperative phase II, two personnel, and one should be an RN. For phase III and discharge, one RN (note that this phase occurs beyond the OR and is associated with inpatient status).
- Confirm that no visitors or HCIRs are in the surgical suite until the patient is prepped and draped for the procedure unless otherwise needed by the surgical team or surgeon.

[ ] **ALERT!**

Limit all traffic within the surgical suite to only those who need to be present for the case. Limiting activity reduces the risk of surgical site infection (SSI).

[ ] **NURSING PEARL**

To ensure a high level of quality and standard of care, the circulator must always be an RN and work within the standard of practice identified by the state board of nursing, in accordance with facility policy and Association of periOperative Registered Nurses (AORN) recommendations for practice.

Evaluate and Ensure

The perioperative RN will evaluate and ensure as follows:

- Evaluate the credentials of the surgical team and the HCIR to determine whether each meets the credentialing requirements for the case and facility, respectively. ▶

Evaluate and Ensure (*continued*)

- Ensure the following sterile field management activities are maintained in collaboration with all surgical team members: Check all items on the sterile field are considered sterile; properly place all items on the sterile field so that they will be subject to minimal movement during the procedure; properly test all equipment before use to prevent unnecessary delays in the case; prevent manipulation of sterile items by placing items in a specific place during setup; plan ahead the position of function for C-arm, laser, or microscope; place items as close to the area where they will be used as possible; secure cords and cables to prevent slippage in the sterile field; and work to prevent clutter on and off the sterile field.

- Promote a culture of safety by acting as follows: Encourage honesty; encourage team members to speak up when errors are present; engage in conflict resolution processes to improve relationships; enhance collaboration through effective communication and shared governance; foster a learning culture; maintain and foster adequate leadership and staffing ratios; and promote behaviors that are respectful and blameless and that improve teamwork.

- If applicable, ensure the following related to the HCIR's presence in the case: Appropriate surgical attire and an identification badge are worn; individual is not in direct contact with the patient or the patient's medical record; instrumentation and any loaned equipment are approved by the healthcare organization and comply with the manufacturer's terminal sterilization guidelines; participation is based on hospital/organization policy and procedure; patient is made aware of the staff members on the surgical team, including the HCIR; patient's dignity, privacy, safety, and confidentiality are safeguarded at all times; and requirement for the individual to be in the room is determined by the nature of the procedure, the surgeon, and the staff (instrument assembly and calibration) and is in compliance with accreditation requirements and local, state, and federal regulations.

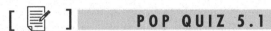

[📝]   POP QUIZ 5.1

The orthopedic surgeon requests that one of the nursing assistive personnel scrubs in to hold retraction on the knee during a right total knee arthroplasty. What should the nurse do?

MANAGEMENT OF PERSONNEL AND SERVICES

The following are the RN's goals for managing personnel and services in the perioperative suite:

- Encourage safety through appropriate staffing. AORN recommends the following parameters for surgical procedure staffing: A minimum of one perioperative RN should be dedicated to performing in the surgical procedure. The perioperative RN supervises, evaluates, and delegates tasks using clinical reasoning skills. The perioperative staffing policy should identify the number of nursing personnel needed by the case based on the complexity of the procedure, team member competencies, patient acuity, monitoring needs, evidence of trauma, and the use of other complex technologies. The staffing plan should include provisions for unplanned, urgent, or emergent procedures and not require the RN to work for more than 12 consecutive hr in a 24-hr period. Staffing level should be set to limit traffic within the perioperative suite.

- Limit the number of personnel in the perioperative suite to only those directly associated with the surgical case.

- Maintain the surgical schedule. Turnover time is the time from the patient leaving the surgical suite to the time of the next patient's arrival. The first case of the day is defined as the time when the first patient scheduled for the OR suite enters the room. Achieving minimal turnover time reduces costs and delays. Surgeon time is associated with the time that the surgeon of record is in the room. Total case time extends from the time set-up in the room for the case to begin until cleanup is complete. ▶

MANAGEMENT OF PERSONNEL AND SERVICES (*continued*)

- Maintain patient confidentiality.
- Promote effective communication among the members of the interdisciplinary team.
- Reduce the risk of infection to the patient.
- Reduce the risk of safety issues associated with the movement of patients and equipment.
- Reduce costs associated with providing services to the patient through the following steps: Open only those necessary sterile supplies, devices, medications, and implants confirmed with the surgeon; regularly review physician preference lists, procedural packs, instrument sets, and other equipment sets to remove items that are not used; and standardize waste management processes.

[UNFOLDING SCENARIO 5A]

The general surgeon arranges with the OR manager to have a medical resident observe a laparoscopic cholecystectomy. The circulator asks the visitor the following questions:

- Have you observed in the OR before?
  - The resident states that this is their first time observing.
- Have you eaten today?
  - The resident states that they just had lunch.
- Do you have to go to the restroom?
  - The resident states that they visited the restroom after lunch.

The circulating nurse escorts the resident to a position in the OR suite where they can see the monitors clearly and be out of the traffic perimeter set by the team. The time-out is called by the circulating nurse, at which point the resident moves closer to the sterile field.

Question

What is the circulating nurse's next step?

[UNFOLDING SCENARIO 5B]

The general surgeon makes the initial incision and inserts the trocars. Insufflation of the abdomen begins. The circulator scans the suite and notices that the resident is swaying back and forth.

Question

What is the circulating nurse's next step?

Assess

- Assess room preparation: For the case cart, assign or delegate an appropriate staff member to check the case carts against the surgeon's preference list and the procedures scheduled for the surgical suite; develop a consistent process related to the way case supplies (materials, instruments, and equipment for the case) are pulled; and evaluate the surgeon's preference list for completeness and identify the needs for upcoming cases. For equipment, assign or delegate an appropriate staff member to gather equipment, minimize the need to move equipment from room to room, and use a standardized list of equipment for the surgical suite where feasible. ▶

Assess (*continued*)

■ Assess personnel staffing assigned to the case: Assign or delegate float staff to assist with the turnover of the room, opening cases, providing breaks, and working to support the case from the sterile core. Utilize assistive personnel to aid in the movement of equipment.

Confirm

■ Confirm that the following key measures are observed before, during, and after the case: Consolidate the back table and organize contents for ease of removal at the end of the case (scrub nurse or technician); keep the OR suite organized (circulating nurse); notify the postanesthesia recovery unit (or the intensive care unit) of the needs of the patient related to a bed and special equipment; notify the environmental services team at the end of the case to expedite turnover of the suite; and prevent contamination by observing the team to ensure that clean surgical attire and personal protective equipment (PPE) are worn within the surgical suite during the opening of a case.

Evaluate and Ensure

The perioperative RN will evaluate and ensure the following:

■ Evaluate the chain of command of members within the interdisciplinary team according to the following standards: Level of the scope of practice for each member working within the environment and the organizational chart hierarchy.

■ Ensure the OR staffing plan includes the following: Provisions for staffing in the event of unplanned, emergent, and urgent procedures; RNs who have not been in direct patient care for more than 12 consecutive hr in a 24-hr period or more than 60 hr in a 7-day work week; strategies to minimize extended work hr related to on-call needs; and use of patient acuity and nursing workload guidelines for the delivery of safe patient care and the promotion of safety within the work environment.

■ Ensure delegation is performed in a manner that takes into consideration the scope of practice for each assistive support member of the interdisciplinary team.

[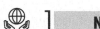]   **NURSING PEARL**

AORN created the perioperative efficiency tool kit to educate perioperative nurses on ways to improve preoperative preparation, reduce delays in surgical start times, and improve operational efficiency associated with the workflow from the sterile processing department through the activities in the OR.

[ ]   **POP QUIZ 5.2**

Following the assessment of the patient's chart for the presence of history and physical examination, as well as consents for surgery, anesthesia, blood transfusion, and laboratory results, a patient is transported to the OR for a right total hip arthroplasty. The anesthesia personnel induce the patient, and the surgical site is prepped. The scrub person is gathering sterile drapes to begin draping the patient. The HCIR is in the suite walking around the sterile field. What is the circulating nurse's next step?

■ Ensure that the perioperative efficiency tool kit, created by AORN in 2016, is followed to establish effective patient and equipment flow as listed as follows in the order of occurrence: Consent and documentation are complete; assessment is performed; patient care and positioning needs are addressed; patient arrival to the OR is not delayed and occurs according to the preset OR schedule; the patient is positioned promptly and in a safe manner; assistance is provided to the anesthesia personnel during induction; setup of room continues until the time-out process begins; assistance is provided to the anesthesia personnel during the patient's emergence from anesthesia; equipment and items to be sterilized are promptly transported to their respective areas for cleaning and sterilization; cleaning of the perioperative suite occurs swiftly to encourage a prompt turnover; and the patient is safely transported to the recovery unit according to facility policy and by at least two members of the surgical team (e.g., anesthesiologist, certified RN anesthetist, or the circulating nurse).

CONFLICT MANAGEMENT

- The OR is a stressful and isolated department in a hospital setting. Isolation is maintained because the area is kept clean and without clutter in the peripheral areas and sterile within the actual surgical suites. The staff must change into standardized clothes before their entry into this area. This area is prone to the incidence and occurrence of disruptive behaviors and interpersonal conflict.
- The following are the key points of concern related to disruptive behaviors: occurrence of incident, person(s) perpetrating the incident, nursing perceptions related to impaired clinical decision-making after experiencing disruptive behaviors, and patient safety errors related to disruptive behaviors.
- Conflict management is an ongoing process in the perioperative environment. The effective management of conflict includes the following steps: Meet face to face with the people involved in the conflict; avoid a blaming culture and cultivate one that promotes learning; encourage an environment of collaboration and communication among team members; and improve work environment continuity through reduction of distractions and avoidance of negative behaviors.

Assess

- Assess the type and level of incivility present in the work environment, including downward violence or disruptive behaviors and lateral violence.
- Assess root causes associated with workplace conflict, including embedded hierarchies, fatigue, ineffective communication, role confusion, stress related to the type of work and challenging procedures, and workload.

Confirm

Confirm that the following measures are taken:

- Encourage the promotion of respect and collaboration among team members.
- Foster learning within the environment.
- Hold team members accountable for behaviors and actions.
- Observe patient safety goals.
- Promote shared decision-making.
- Reduce barriers to effective communication.

[ ]   **ALERT!**

Establishing a blame-free and patient-centered safety culture is a systems-level intervention that improves patient care and outcomes.

Evaluate and Ensure

- Evaluate the situation and whether workplace violence prevention programs are available at the facility.
- Evaluate and consider the following course of action related to incivility, conflict management, and the promotion of a healthy workplace: Assess one's own actions related to incivility; engage in ongoing training related to conflict management and healthy workplace promotion; remain aware

[ ]   **POP QUIZ 5.3**

The orthopedic surgeon asks the HCIR to get the new bone cement that they had talked about earlier in the day. The circulating nurse alerts the surgeon that the cement has not gone through the appropriate approvals for use according to facility policy. A conflict arises between the surgeon and the nurse, with the surgeon insisting on using the cement. What should the circulating nurse do?

of environmental controls and policies that exist to prevent and reduce conflict and violent incidents; report issues using a standardized reporting protocol and system and in accordance with facility policy and procedure; take action to initiate change and deescalate the situation if possible; and understand the importance of becoming aware of threatening situations and potential for violence. ▶

Evaluate and Ensure (*continued*)

■ Ensure active participation in conflict reduction in the workplace by adhering to the following provisions in the American Nurses Association Code of Ethics: engaging in continuous improvement activities that foster team collaboration and communication, participating in postevent meetings, providing support to team members, and utilizing counseling resources at the facility.

VISITORS

The perioperative nurse is charged with supervising all visitors in the surgical suite. The presence of visitors in the surgical suite should be limited.

Assess

Assess the following associated with visitors to the surgical suite:

■ Approval for visitation granted by leadership
■ Need for access to other personnel (e.g., HCIR and the scrub personnel)
■ Position in the suite
■ Presence of appropriate scrub attire, personal protective equipment, and a facility-approved identification badge
■ Prior experience of presence in the OR
■ Reason for presence in the suite

[⚙]   **ALERT!**

In some facilities, the visitor may need to have an approval signed by the patient. The perioperative nurse should adhere to the facility policy on visitors in the surgical suite.

Confirm

■ Confirm that the patient has been made aware that there will be visitors in the surgical suite and the reason for their presence.
■ Confirm that all visitors understand that all patient information is to be kept confidential, and there should be no physical movement during the time-out process.
■ Confirm that visitors have eaten before being in the room and that they know what to do if they feel faint.

Evaluate and Ensure

■ Evaluate the suite routinely to ensure that movement within the area is limited, noise is reduced, and traffic is kept to a minimum.
■ Ensure the following safety and traffic control interventions are implemented: Create signage indicating specific safety guidelines to be observed (e.g., laser in use, isolation case, latex allergy); develop language to be used for nonessential visitors

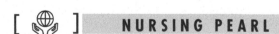

[🤲]   **NURSING PEARL**

The nurse is the first line of defense for patients. Remaining vigilant in one's advocacy for patients and their safety is a top priority.

when asking them to leave the suite; educate visitors on the appropriate exit and entry areas (e.g., limit access to the sterile core); and protect the sterile field from contamination and compromise by setting a clear perimeter for visitors to walk around.

RESOURCES

American Nurses Association. (2015). *American Nurses Association position statement on incivility, bullying, and workplace violence.* https://www.nursingworld.org/~49d6e3/globalassets/practiceandpolicy/nursing -excellence/incivility-bullying-and-workplace-violence--ana-position-statement.pdf

Association of periOperative Registered Nurses. (2013). Recommended practices for maintaining a sterile field. In *Perioperative standards and recommended* practices. Author.

Association of periOperative Registered Nurses. (2016). *AORN perioperative efficiency tool kit* [Toolkit]. https:// www.aorn.org/-/media/aorn/guidelines/tool-kits/perioperative-efficiency/aorn-perioperative-efficiency-tool -kit-webinar.pdf?la=en

Association of periOperative Registered Nurses. (2018). Guideline for a safe environment of care. In Guidelines for *perioperative practice*. Author.

Association of periOperative Registered Nurses. (2019a). AORN position statement on perioperative registered nurse circulator dedicated to every patient undergoing an operative or other invasive procedure. In Guidelines *for perioperative practice*. Author.

Association of periOperative Registered Nurses. (2019b). *Guideline essentials: Key takeaways.* https://www.aorn .org/essentials/team-communication

Association of periOperative Registered Nurses. (2020a). AORN position statement on allied health care providers and support personnel in the perioperative practice setting. In Guidelines for perioperative practice. Author.

Association of periOperative Registered Nurses. (2020b). AORN position statement on perioperative safe staffing and on-call practices. In Guidelines for perioperative practice. Author.

Association of periOperative Registered Nurses. (2020c). AORN position statement on the role of the health care industry representative in perioperative settings. In Guidelines for perioperative practice. Author.

Association of periOperative Registered Nurses. (2021). *Re-entry guidance for health care facilities and medical device representatives.* https://www.aorn.org/guidelines/aorn-support/re-entry-guidance-for-health-care-facilities

Link, T. (2018). Guideline implementation: Team communication. *AORN Journal, 108*(2), 165–177. https://doi.org/ 10.1002/aorn.12300

Mews, P. A., & Wafer, P. (2020). *Perioperative efficiency: Patient safety, workflow, and quality. AORN: Safe surgery together toolkit.* Association of periOperative Registered Nurses.

Norton, B., & Mordas, D. (2018). A postprocedure wrap-up tool for improving OR communication and performance. *AORN Journal, 107*(1), 108–115. https://doi.org/10.1002/aorn.12007

6 COMMUNICATION AND DOCUMENTATION

OVERVIEW

- Creating a patient safety culture requires effective team collaboration and communication. Written communication through documentation also aids in safeguarding the patient while promoting effective and efficient care. This chapter emphasizes the following aspects of perioperative nursing: effective hand-off protocols and documentation to facilitate communication, workflow, and patient safety; employment of methods to enhance quality; promotion of respect among team members; and the role of education in developing a patient safety culture.
- Throughout each phase of the perioperative experience, the nurse will perform duties using the ACE process: **A**ssess, **C**onfirm, and **E**valuate and **E**nsure.

COMMUNICATION AMONG CAREGIVERS

- Communication among caregivers in the perioperative setting is vital to maintaining the safety of patients and staff and reducing barriers to team collaboration.
- Communication issues have been identified as a root cause for sentinel events that occur during surgery and range from wrong-patient and wrong-site events to wrong-procedure events that cause harm to the patient.

Assess

Assess the following potential communication barriers:

- High noise levels within the perioperative suite
- Impediments to exchange of dialogue due to equipment or layout of the surgical suite
- Irrelevant conversation among the team members
- Nonessential activity or movement (during time-out, critical conversations between team members, induction, emergence, counting, and specimen handling)
- Patient's language barriers or nonverbal status

Confirm

- Confirm that the members of the perioperative team maintain a patient safety culture through the following strategies: accountability for behaviors in the OR suite; adequacy of staffing; adherence to the pillars of safety (trust, report, and improve); appreciation of members' contributions to the team; attentiveness and cessation of all activity during the time-out; commitment to voicing safety concerns; encouragement of honesty; and promotion of a learning culture. ▶

[ ]   **ALERT!**

Speaking up can save lives. Encourage a culture of safety for everyone.

Confirm (*continued*)

■ Confirm that the following information is communicated to the interdisciplinary healthcare team members involved in the patient's care: communication needs of the patient, implants or implanted device location, medications used during surgery, report of allergies, and status of the patient's medical condition during and at the end of surgery (e.g., breaks in sterility, fluid losses, blood loss, and urine output).

Evaluate and Ensure

■ Evaluate potential and actual system failures that undermine a culture of safety associated with the surgical team, including deviation from standards of practice or errors in practice, interpersonal conflicts, lapses in judgment, and mistakes in practice.

■ Ensure effective communication and collaboration by doing the following: Address behaviors that could lead to harm of the patient or create barriers in the work environment; ensure that a standardized briefing process, known as the *Universal Protocol*, is used during each of the operative phases; ensure adequate staff is available to move the patient at the end of the procedure; monitor and cross-check processes and procedures used in practice; read back and verify when needing clarity, receiving critical information on a patient, dispensing medications or fluids to the field by the circulator to the scrub nurse, and receiving medication or other orders from the surgeon or anesthesiologist; use clear, specific, and concise descriptions of tasks to be delegated or needs of the case; use the chain of command and standardized process when reporting issues; and use a standardized process, tools, and chain of command when reporting patient information related to adverse event issues, needing a team debriefing at the end of a procedure or after an adverse event, transferring care to the receiving unit (e.g., PACU, ICU), transferring care to relief staff, and voicing concerns as they arise.

[ ]   NURSING PEARL

Communication is one of the most vital components of a nurse's toolbox. Use effective communication to promote team collaboration, reduce incivility in the work environment, and improve patient outcomes.

[ ]   POP QUIZ 6.1

A 50-year-old male is transported to the OR from the preoperative holding area to undergo an arteriovascular graft for dialysis. The graft product is opened without verifying the expiration. The circulating nurse notices that the product is expired just prior to the surgeon inserting the graft. The circulating nurse alerts the surgeon that the product is expired. What could have prevented this error?

[UNFOLDING SCENARIO 6A]

A 58-year-old metal worker enters the OR for the removal of a mass in their left upper scapular area under general anesthesia. The patient's history and physical examination review reveals that there is a 40-year history of smoking, chronic obstructive pulmonary disease (COPD), and hypertension. The patient's height is documented as 70 in, and the weight is 265 lb.

The patient is not yet sedated and is able to move onto the OR bed and lie in the supine position. The anesthesia provider confers with the surgeon on whether the patient should be positioned in the right lateral position to maintain the compromised airway. The surgeon responds, "Sure," and leaves it to the scrub person. The anesthesia provider begins induction with assistance from the circulating nurse.

(continued)

The circulating nurse then gathers the pillows and axillary roll and stands by the patient's side while loosening the safety strap. The anesthesia provider helps the circulating nurse shift the patient to lie on their right side with the knees bent until comfortable and with the right arm extended on an arm board. The nurse places the axillary roll under the right shoulder area and places a pillow between the legs and under the left elbow, which is resting on a Mayo stand. The safety strap is placed over the patient's thighs and attached to the OR table. The circulator confirms with the anesthesia provider that the patient is in a good position.

The circulating nurse proceeds with the prep; there is a little pooling of the iodine-based solution, but because the procedure is so short, the circulator leaves it. After draping is finished, the circulating nurse helps the scrub person move the Mayo stand for additional sterile draping by the scrub person. The scrub person lays the patient's arm on the left side of the body to rest while the Mayo stand is draped, and the back table is repositioned by the scrub person to the left of the surgeon and the incision site. The left arm is then positioned on the sterile-draped Mayo stand.

The circulator calls for the time-out and reads the checklist. All items on the checklist are approved by the team except for allergies. The anesthesia personnel reminds the team that the patient has an allergy to iodine. The case is short, and the surgeon cleans the area around the left upper scapula with sterile saline.

The circulating nurse begins documentation on the electronic health record. Suddenly, the patient's legs slip from the table, the surgeon yells, and contents from the Mayo stand fall. The anesthesia provider removes the drapes to hold the patient and prevent them from slipping down the table. One side of the safety strap had not been securely fastened. The anesthesia provider also notices a rash present on the area of the prepped skin.

Question 1

What errors in communication occurred?

Question 2

How could the injury to the patient have been prevented?

DOCUMENTATION IN THE PATIENT RECORD

The legal health record consists of the documentation of all services, products used for service, medications, plans of care (assessment, diagnosis, planning, implementation, and evaluation), and notes on end-of-life support decisions and advance directives related to patient care.

Assess

- Assess the patient care record for the following: Complete an accurate informed consent for surgery and anesthesia administration, including the date (typically must be dated fewer than 30 days prior but depends on facility policy), name of the healthcare facility, invasive procedure to be performed, and healthcare representative performing the procedure, signatures with date and time of the patient and healthcare provider's signature (if patient is unable to sign, signature of legal patient representative), and statement of the risks and benefits associated with the proposed procedure and alternatives to the procedure; disposition orders for the placenta for live births (facility dependent) and death certificate documentation in the case of fetal demise; disposition of limb documentation (for amputation); history and physical report (within the last 30 days or according to facility policy); laboratory and radiology reports; medication records; orders pertaining to the planned procedure; and other documentation associated with the procedure (e.g., limb disposal consents, blood transfusion consent).
- Assess equipment settings and document initial settings and all changes to settings during the procedure for ablation equipment, argon-enhanced coagulation, arthroscopic irrigation equipment, autoclaves, defibrillators, electrosurgical generator, fluid warmers, hysteroscopy pumps, infusion pumps, lasers, light sources, medical gas (e.g., nitrogen), microscopes, patient warming devices (forced-warm air), pneumatic tourniquets, and sequential compression devices.

Confirm

- Confirm that the perioperative record includes documentation of the following according to facility policy and procedure: notes associated with adverse events or unplanned activities as per facility policy (e.g., retained foreign body, injury to the patient, change from a laparoscopic procedure to an open procedure); products used during the procedure (including implantable material); record of explants, implants, and surgical specimens; roles, credentials, and the time present in the perioperative suite for a healthcare industry representative (HCIR), law enforcement, observers, perioperative personnel, pathology and radiology staff, support staff, and surgeons and assistants; time associated with administration of antibiotics, transfer of specimens from the surgical field to pathology, removal of specimens from the surgical field and fixative times (if needed), surgical start and end, time-out process, placement of tourniquet and settings, and transport of patient into and out of the surgical suite.

[UNFOLDING SCENARIO 6B]

The case of the 58-year-old metal worker who needed a removal of a mass in their left upper scapular area under general anesthesia has ended, and the patient has been extubated. The circulating nurse and the nurse anesthetist make final adjustments to the patient's position to transfer to the hospital bed. The circulating nurse reassesses the rash and notes that the area is still red.

Question

The circulating nurse finalizes documentation on the electronic health record. What information should the nurse include on the chart?

Evaluate and Ensure

- Evaluate barriers to communication among healthcare team members. Environmental factors include interruptions in the surgical process, multiple conversations, music, and noise. Human factors include disruptive behavior, embedded hierarchies, fatigue, focus on a specific patient issue or surgical issue, hunger, and stress.
- Evaluate the documentation tools used in perioperative practice and the downtime process associated with documentation offline.
- Evaluate documentation to ensure compliance with state guidelines and national accreditation requirements related to the following areas: blood and tissue tracking, implant tracking, infection control practices (e.g., surgical preparation methods and antibiotic prophylaxis), injury reduction measures (e.g., positioning aids used), intraoperative testing, medication administration and reconciliation, pain management interventions, patient education (preoperative phase), and urinary catheter insertion.
- Ensure that the patient's health record is safeguarded for privacy using the following procedures: Limit the use of mobile devices in the perioperative suite; minimize the electronic record on the computer screen to restrict access to the patient record during the procedure; observe guidelines related to the Health Insurance Portability and Accountability Act (HIPAA) of 1996; protect the paper health record by covering all patient information; refrain from sharing facility-assigned log-in information with other staff and visitors to the OR unit or individual suite; retain all patient care-related information in its original and legally reproducible format according to facility policy; and use the facility-approved platform to access the patient's health record.
- Ensure all pertinent information is documented in the electronic health record or paper chart.
- Ensure that the facility policy related to documentation is followed.
- Ensure communication processes are followed to support continuity of patient care, such as by using one of the following procedures.
- *IPASS the BATON*: This type of hand-off procedure requires the following information be shared when transferring care to another healthcare provider: *Introduction* of the staff to the patient; *Patient name*, identifiers, age, sex, and location of the surgery; *Assessment* of vital signs, focused assessment related to surgery; *Situation* or circumstances that led to the patient having surgery; *Safety* concerns associated with critical lab results, allergies, and positioning; *Background information* associated with comorbidities, medications, family, and social history; *Actions* that will need to be taken to ensure positive patient outcome; *Timing* of actions and the urgency level associated with the surgery; *Ownership* of the roles and responsibilities for each aspect of care during the perioperative experience; and *Next or anticipated changes* and the plan for the surgical team to provide care. ▶

[ ] NURSING PEARL

An old adage states that, "If you did not document it, you did not do it." Remember to document all activities and actions that occur before and during the procedure and upon transfer to the post-anesthesia care unit (PACU).

[ ] ALERT!

Tissue Tracking

The Joint Commission (TJC) recommends that all staff members coming into contact with any type of tissue, bones, or vessels be tracked and that this tracking be documented according to U.S. Food and Drug Administration (FDA) and American Association of Tissue Banks (AATB) requirements.

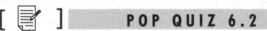

[ ] POP QUIZ 6.2

A patient is transported to the OR from the medical–surgical floor to undergo a right total hip arthroplasty. Once the patient is positioned on the surgical table, the nurse notices erythema and swelling of the right heel not reported during hand-off communication upon the patient's transfer to the OR. What should the nurse do first?

Evaluate and Ensure (*continued*)

- *SBAR:* This widely known hand-off procedure identifies the four aspects of information needed when reporting off to a relief nurse or another level of care. In perioperative nursing, SBAR is used as follows: *Situation:* summarizes the situation at a given point in time (i.e., count results at the end of the surgery, status of dressing application, documentation requirements); *Background:* describes issues that may have occurred during the procedure (contamination of an instrument, person, table, etc.); *Assessment:* describes how well the patient tolerated the procedure and if there are special considerations (drain placement, tourniquet time, etc.); *Recommendation:* describes other recommendations for patient care issues that still need attention or require follow-up in the surgical suite.
- *Read Back and Verify:* This procedure requires all perioperative personnel to read back and verify (audibly for all team members) orders from the surgeon and/or delegated tasks, including deviations from the normal standard of care (e.g., trauma cases, emergencies, disasters); medications dispensed to the sterile field; positioning of the patient; specimen handling, labeling, documentation, and transport (e.g. tissue, blood, fluid); and verbal orders from the surgeon or anesthesiologist.
- *Standardized Surgical Checklist:* This checklist is used during the preprocedure check-in, patient sign-in to the surgical suite, time-out, and patient sign-out of the surgical suite and transport to the next level of care.
- Ensure that the documentation associated with tissue tracking is complete and the process adheres to facility, state, and federal guidelines (Table 6.1).
- Ensure that the documentation associated with implants is complete and the process adheres to facility, state, and federal guidelines.
- Ensure the following information is obtained related to autologous tissue according to facility policy: date of recovery, disposition of the tissue and all those who handle it, name of the surgeon, type of procedure, type of storage and temperature, and type of tissue and method of preservation.

TABLE 6.1 Tissue Tracking Recommendations and Guidelines		
TISSUE TYPE	**STORAGE**	**SPECIAL CONSIDERATIONS**

Cranial bone flaps	Frozen, cryopreserved, or in a subcutaneous pocket for replantation	• Facility guidelines should include the method for preparing the bone flap:
		  ○ Removal of blood and excess tissue
		  ○ Use of a low-linting sterile material to dry the bone
		  ○ Use of the sterile technique to prepare the bone for packaging

Femoral head	Can be stored in the iliac pocket	• The storage and preservation of the femoral head in the iliac pocket is associated with total hip arthroplasty revision procedures.
Parathyroid tissue	Cryopreserved or auto-transplanted	• Call ahead to pathology when the tissue is in transit. • Place the specimen in a sterile specimen cup and on sterile ice. • Transport the specimen to the pathology lab as soon as possible.
Skin	Preserved or auto-transplanted (i.e., split-thickness graft)	• Preserve the skin through refrigeration according to facility policy and guidelines. • Place the graft on a sheet of tulle gras with the epithelial side down. • Wrap the graft in moistened saline gauze or place it in a sterile container.
Vessels	Preserved or transplanted	• Store in a buffered storage solution or tissue culture medium for no longer than 14 days.

RESOURCES

Agency for Healthcare Research and Quality. (2019, June). *Team STEPPS 2.0.* U.S. Department of Health and Human Services, Agency for Healthcare Research and Quality. https://www.ahrq.gov/teamstepps/instructor/index.html

American Health Information Management Association. (2011, February). Fundamentals of the legal health record and designated record set. *Journal of AHIMA, 82*(2). https://library.ahima.org/doc?oid=104008#.YG9bNuhKiUk

American Nurses Association. (2015). *American Nurses Association position statement on incivility, bullying, and workplace violence.* https://www.nursingworld.org/~49d6e3/globalassets/practiceandpolicy/nursing-excellence/incivility-bullying-and-workplace-violence--ana-position-statement.pdf

Association of periOperative Registered Nurses. (2019). Autologous tissue management. In *Guidelines for perioperative practice.* Author.

Association of periOperative Registered Nurses. (2020a). Information management. In *Guidelines for perioperative practice.* Author.

Association of periOperative Registered Nurses. (2020b). Team communication. In *Guidelines for perioperative practice.* Author.

Link, T. (2018). Guideline implementation: Team communication. *AORN Journal, 108*(2), 165–177. https://doi.org/10.1002/aorn.12300

Norton, B., & Mordas, D. (2018). A postprocedure wrap-up tool for improving OR communication and performance. *AORN Journal, 107*(1), 108–115. https://doi.org/10.1002/aorn.12007

Pradetha, A. (2017, October 9). Meeting Joint Commission tissue tracking requirements. *Mobile Aspects.* https://www.mobileaspects.com/meeting-joint-commission-tissue-tracking-requirements

7 INFECTION PREVENTION AND CONTROL OF ENVIRONMENT, INSTRUMENTATION, AND SUPPLIES

OVERVIEW

- Regulatory and accrediting organizations have stringent requirements around infection prevention, and facilities have mechanisms to prevent infection, but hospital-acquired infections (HAIs) remain high.
- According to The Joint Commission (TJC), the incidence of surgical site infections (SSIs), one type of HAI, is staggering, with approximately 500,000 cases reported annually.
- Throughout each phase of the perioperative experience, the nurse will perform duties using the ACE process: Assess, Confirm, and Evaluate and Ensure.

REGULATORY STANDARDS FOR INFECTION PREVENTION

- The *Guideline for Prevention of Surgical Site Infection* was first published in 1999 by a team of medical doctors and infection control practitioners.
- Healthcare professionals followed these guidelines inconsistently. In response, a national quality improvement standardization project led to the development of the Surgical Care Improvement Project (SCIP), a collaboration of the Centers for Medicare and Medicaid Services (CMS) and the Centers for Disease Control and Prevention (CDC). Several SCIP elements focus on preventing SSIs.
- TJC expanded upon these guidelines to develop National Patient Safety Goals (NPSGs). Specifically, NPSG.07.05.01, *Implement Evidence-Based Practices for Preventing Surgical Site Infections*, specifies standards of practice to prevent SSIs in OR suites, ambulatory care centers, and office-based surgery centers.
- The American College of Surgeons National Surgery Quality Improvement Program provides guidance and analyses on quality improvement processes for participating hospitals.

Assess

- Assess compliance with federal, state, and local regulatory bodies related to infection prevention associated with sharps handling, single-use and reusable products, skin preparation, surgical antibiotic prophylaxis, surgical gloves, urinary catheter use, thermoregulation, and surgical smoke evacuation.
- Assess facility policy and procedures associated with the prevention of SSI.

Confirm

- Confirm that all members of the surgical team are compliant with and adhere to TJC guidelines outlined in the annually updated NPSGs. ▶

Confirm (*continued*)

- Confirm that the Occupational Safety and Health Administration (OSHA), CDC, and TJC regulatory standards and Association of periOperative Registered Nurses (AORN) professional guidelines associated with infection prevention practices for each of the following are maintained. Blood glucose levels as follows: cardiac patient—less than 180 mg/dL; preoperative phase—less than 200 mg/dL; perioperative phase—between 110 and 150 mg/dL. Nasal decolonization for patients undergoing cardiothoracic, spine, and orthopedic procedures or as indicated by the facility policy; normothermia throughout the surgical procedure with a core temperature above 95°F (35°C); and sharps handling and injury prevention. Skin preparation before the surgical procedure should be done according to facility policy, using single-use barrier products, surgical antibiotic prophylaxis, surgical gloves, and surgical smoke toxicity.

[ ]   ALERT!

In 2021, multiple states (Illinois, Oregon, Kentucky, Rhode Island, Colorado) passed legislation mandating the use of surgical smoke evacuation.

Evaluate and Ensure

- Evaluate the perioperative environment for any potential sources of infection.
- Ensure adherence to AORN guidelines for transmission-based precautions as follows: Reduce the transmission of bioburden and microbial contamination that may enter the surgical site through the patient's skin, surgical personnel, air, and contaminated surfaces or instrumentation; use standard precautions when providing patient care; use contact precautions with patients with known infections or those who are colonized with a pathogen; and wear the appropriate personal protective equipment (PPE) during all patient handling and if it is anticipated that there will be exposure to blood-borne pathogens, infectious material, or bodily fluids.

[UNFOLDING SCENARIO 7A]

The sterile field is prepped and draped for a dual procedure, an open cholecystectomy and exploratory laparotomy. The scrub personnel establish a neutral zone. During the procedure, the surgeon makes the incision to start the procedure and inadvertently pierces the drape with the knife blade.

Question

What is the purpose of a neutral zone? What should the scrub personnel do in this scenario?

SURGICAL SCRUBBING AND HAND HYGIENE

- Colonization is the asymptomatic carrying of organisms on the skin, in the body fluids, or on the tissues, not causing a clinically adverse effect for an individual.
- Decolonization is the use of antimicrobial or antiseptic agents to suppress or eradicate colonization.
- Perioperative personnel must adhere to strict hand hygiene practices when providing patient care and handling sterile supplies and equipment. This section discusses surgical scrubbing techniques and hand hygiene practices to be followed in the perioperative area.
- Surgical scrubbing uses surgical skin antiseptics to minimize resident flora on the skin, reducing the risk of contamination by microorganisms during operative or invasive procedures.

Assess

- Assess the use of appropriate hand antisepsis by all members of the surgical team: broad spectrum, fast acting, U.S. Food and Drug Administration (FDA) approved, and persistent in maintaining the reduction of bacterial colonization at 6 hr.
- Assess the use of appropriate techniques and solutions, noting that alcohol-based solutions cannot penetrate spores, and mechanical friction during soap and water handwashing is most effective against spore-forming organisms such as *Clostridium difficile*, *Bacillus anthracis*, and norovirus.
- Assess decolonization protocols, including the following: Evaluate allergies and sensitivities to skin antiseptics; remove all visible soil and debris from the surgical site using an approved skin antiseptic agent; use intranasal administration of mupirocin in combination with an FDA-approved skin antiseptic agent such as Chlorhexidine gluconate (CHG) for decolonization; hair should be left at the surgical site unless it is clinically contraindicated; and instruct patients to bathe or shower with either soap and water or the prescribed skin antisepsis.

Confirm

- Perioperative personnel should confirm that the following hand hygiene goals are met: Maintain healthy skin; maintain healthy nails; maintain short nails, length not exceeding 2 mm (0.08 in.), to decrease the risk of bacterial colonization beneath the nail, prevent perforation of the surgical gloves, and revent patient injury during transfer; use alcohol-based hand scrub; use facility-approved moisturizers that are compatible with hand hygiene products to prevent degradation of scrub solutions and breakdown of surgical gloves; use water that is in the temperature range of 70°F to 80°F (21°C–26.7°C); wash hands with soap and water for a minimum of 15 seconds.

 ALERT!

Perioperative personnel must do the following:

- Perform a proper surgical hand scrub as the first line of defense in minimizing pathogens' transmission from the hands to the patient.
- Provide a second line of defense by donning sterile gloves to decrease the risk of SSI.

Evaluate and Ensure

- Evaluate the skin integrity of those who are performing a surgical scrub before the procedure. Personnel with visibly cracked or peeling skin should refrain from scrubbing in for the procedure. Personnel with subcutaneous outbreaks or skin abrasions are less likely to perform appropriate hand hygiene.

 ALERT!

Artificial nails have been implicated in the spread of gram-negative bacteria and yeast.

- Ensure that the surgical hand scrub (alcohol-based or packaged scrub brush) is performed per the manufacturer's instructions for use (IFU) and according to AORN standards for hand hygiene. Don a surgical mask, remove all jewelry from the hands and the wrists, open the scrub brush, turn the water on, remove debris from under the fingernails using the disposable nail, rinse the hands, use the scrub brush to address all four sides of each hand and each finger according to the manufacturer's recommendation for use, hold the hands higher than the elbows during the scrubbing process, avoid splashing water on surgical attire, and rinse the hands by running each arm through the stream in an upward fashion.
- Ensure that perioperative personnel perform hand hygiene for activities including, but not limited to, the following; before and after patient contact, including site marking and wound care, or involving blood or bodily fluids; before and after accessing or handling an invasive device, a vascular device, a urinary catheter, or a colostomy bag; before eating and after using the restroom; and before performing a clean or sterile task or after removing PPE. ▶

Evaluate and Ensure (*continued*)

■ Ensure that perioperative personnel are not wearing artificial nails or polish that may inhibit the ability to properly perform hand hygiene or interfere with the procedure.

■ Ensure that perioperative personnel are encouraged to double-glove so that the outer glove can act as an additional barrier that can be removed to avoid delay caused by hand hygiene. Remove gloves after completing patient care activities and performing hand hygiene. Weigh the risks and benefits of wearing gloves during life-saving interventions such as ventilation and airway management.

[UNFOLDING SCENARIO 7B]

During the procedure, the abdominal cholecystectomy with exploratory laparotomy is taking longer than scheduled, and it is time for the scrub person to have a lunch break. The relief scrub is at the scrub sink getting ready to scrub in. The circulating nurse checks on the relief scrub and notices that only a quick application of the alcohol-based hand antisepsis product has been completed. The circulating nurse is next to be relieved for lunch. The relief nurse comes into the room noting that her hands are dry. She takes lotion out of her pocket brought from home and applies it to her hands.

Question

How should the circulating nurse intervene with the scrub nurse and the relief nurse?

SURGICAL ATTIRE

Surgical attire consists of the facility-approved scrub shirt and pants, the bouffant cap, and shoe covers. At the surgical field, the attire consists of an additional layer of protection including the surgical gown and eye protection. This section reviews specifics associated with AORN's guideline for surgical attire.

Assess

■ Assess the following related to head-to-toe surgical attire requirements: Personal clothing must be nonlinting, covered by approved scrub attire, and laundered daily and when contaminated with blood, bodily fluids, or infectious materials. Arms may be covered with long-sleeved, hospital-laundered jackets when performing the patient's surgical skin prep. The head must be covered when entering semi-restricted and restricted areas to avoid shedding hair and bacteria that may contaminate a sterile field. Jewelry should not be worn. If it is approved to be worn, the following is advised by AORN: Scrubbed personnel must not wear jewelry, and unscrubbed personnel must keep jewelry to a minimum. The face must be covered, and the feet should be protected with shoes that are clean and have closed heels and front.

Confirm

Confirm that surgical scrub attire is laundered properly.

■ Perioperative personnel cannot easily monitor quality and consistency in home laundering and should use the following guidelines: Do not launder surgical scrub attire at home. Do not place contaminated scrubs in a washer, as this may deposit bioburden and transmit microorganisms to other clothing. Do not store surgical scrubs in lockers to wear again. Remove surgical attire before leaving the facility. Wear facility-laundered scrubs washed following state recommendations or CDC guidelines.

Evaluate and Ensure

- Evaluate scrub attire for pilling of fabric, tears, lint, or soiling.
- Ensure that the laundering of surgical attire occurs through an approved vendor selected by the facility.

STANDARD AND TRANSMISSION-BASED PRECAUTIONS

- The CDC identifies two tiers of precautions to be considered when preventing infection in the healthcare setting: standard and transmission-based precautions. Standard precautions, considered the first tier of precautions, are used for all patients, and are used for patients who are infected or colonized with an infectious agent. Transmission-based precautions are the second tier of infection control and are used in addition to standard precautions.
- The goal of using both standard and transmission-based precautions is to prevent infection transmission to healthcare personnel, patients, and visitors in the facility.

Assess

Assess the patient related to the need for the following precautions:

- Standard precautions: Use standard precautions for all patient care. Follow the CDC protocol, which includes donning appropriate PPE, following respiratory hygiene principles, handling and disinfecting patient care equipment and instruments, and performing hand hygiene.
- Contact precautions: Use contact precautions when a patient is known to have Group A Streptococcus (*Streptococcus pyogenes*), known as "flesh-eating bacteria," or multidrug resistant organisms (MDROs).
- Droplet and airborne precautions: Use droplet or airborne precautions for patients with adenovirus, coronaviruses (SARS-CoV, MERS-CoV, and SARS-CoV-2), draining tuberculosis (TB) lesions, Ebola virus, group A Streptococcus infections, smallpox, and varicella-zoster virus.
- Droplet precautions: Use droplet precautions for adenovirus, rhinovirus, group A Streptococcus (*S. pyogenes*), influenza, mumps, *Neisseria meningitides* (meningitis), and pertussis (whooping cough).

Confirm

Confirm that all perioperative personnel don the appropriate PPE associated with each type of precaution according to the CDC (n.d.-a) guidelines:

- Airborne precautions: gloves, particulate respirator (e.g., N95 or powered air purifying respirator)
- Contact precautions: face mask, gloves, gown
- Droplet precautions: face mask, gloves, eye protection (shields, goggles, glasses)

Evaluate and Ensure

- Evaluate the activity within the perioperative suite, both on and off the sterile field, for biohazardous fluid spills and cross-contamination.
- Evaluate patients for the presence of MDRO or other organisms requiring more than standard precautions.

 ALERT!

Perioperative personnel should consider each patient's blood and bodily fluids as contagious.

Sweat and tears are not considered contagious. (CDC, n.d.-b)

Ensure that the hierarchy of controls to prevent the spread of infection is utilized by perioperative personnel, including adherence to policy and procedure for isolation and reducing the transmission of disease, elimination of the hazard, management of environmental controls (e.g., negative pressure for airborne disease), safe work practice (e.g., safe sharps handling, proper body mechanics), and wearing appropriate PPE.

[UNFOLDING SCENARIO 7C]

The surgical case is wrapping up, and final counts are complete. The scrub person begins to remove blades from the handle when a blade slips and slices through both of the gloves on one hand. The circulator calls the charge nurse for an emergency relief scrub.

Question

What should the scrub nurse do?

STANDARDS FOR STERILIZATION OF INSTRUMENTATION

AORN has issued guidelines and standards associated with the sterilization of instrumentation. This section will covers some of the newest guidelines and key points.

Assess

■ Assess all wrapped packaging for tears, rips, moisture, and sterilization indicators.
■ Assess all rigid containers for a proper seal and indication that sterilization parameters have been met.

Confirm

■ Confirm that the guidelines for sterile processing personnel are met.
■ If sterilization parameters have not been met, confirm the following is completed: Assess whether the failure puts the patient at risk, complete an incident report per facility policy, confirm the chemical or biologic indicator results, inform appropriate leadership, investigate the failure, and quarantine potentially affected items.

Evaluate and Ensure

■ Evaluate all packaging and containers to ensure integrity and sterilization before dispensing to the sterile field.
■ Ensure the AORN guidelines for sterile processing are followed. Sterilization processes include items sterilized in designated processing areas, phacoemulsification handpieces in a vertical position, and reusable sterilized semi-critical items. Sterilization, instead of high-level disinfection, is considered more effective in the prevention of transmissible pathogens.
■ Ensure that all perioperative and sterile processing personnel are aware of work hazards and handling of hazardous chemical sterilizers, including ethylene oxide, hydrogen peroxide, and peracetic acid. Know the immediate use steam sterilization (IUSS) process (formerly known as flash sterilization). Follow instructions for rigid container use during the IUSS cycle and only use IUSS cycles when item is for immediate use, terminal sterilization process is not possible, and the device manufacturer provides written instructions for using IUSS related to cleaning, sterilization cycle type, exposure, temperature, and drying parameters. Perform management processes for a wet pack or wet load, including the following: Take corrective action when there is moisture on or in a package, reassess the entire load as moisture on or in a package possibly indicates problems with the sterilizer, steam supply, or load configuration, and resterilize the package. Process reusable medical devices based on how they are intended for use. Store sterile items in controlled conditions. Transport sterile items according to facility policy and with adherence to CDC, FDA, and AORN guidelines. Understand how to use MSDSs in the event of exposure. Use a sterile barrier system to transport all sterile items to the point of use. Use biologic indicators specific to each sterilization process and type of sterilizer. ▶

Evaluate and Ensure (*continued*)

■ Ensure that the instrumentation is returned to its original container or a transport container by disassembling all instruments with removable parts, flushing sterile water through hollow instruments, opening hinged instruments to expose box locks or serrated edges, and separating delicate and small instruments with sharp edges.

[ ]   **ALERT!**

AORN recommends that healthcare organizations do the following:

• Designate only qualified individuals to manage and oversee sterile processing personnel.
• Increase awareness of the environmental impact of the sterilization process.
• Monitor and control the flow of steam to sterilizers.
• Standardize and monitor off-site sterilization processes.

[UNFOLDING SCENARIO 7D]

During the abdominal procedure, the circulating nurse opens the tray for the Bookwalter retractor set. Upon inspection, the nurse notes that the chemical indicator is missing. Only two of these retractor sets are available, and the other one is being used in another case. The surgeon wants the retractor set IUSS to use in this case.

Question

What is the nurse's next course of action?

DOCUMENTATION OF STERILIZATION AND DISINFECTION

The perioperative nurse verifies that documentation of sterilization and disinfection is complete for steam and high-level disinfection. This section reviews AORN's recommendations related to the documentation of sterilization processes.

Assess

■ Assess the IUSS daily and upon each use for appropriate functioning according to the facility policy and procedures.
■ Assess sterilization logs for accuracy and completeness.

Confirm

Confirm that the following documentation requirements are completed related to all methods of sterilization:

■ Contents
■ Exposure parameters
■ Load number
■ Operator's name or initials
■ Results of physical, chemical, and biologic monitors
■ Sterilization records in compliance with the healthcare organization's policies and regulations at the federal, state, and local levels

Evaluate and Ensure

■ Evaluate and ensure that perioperative or sterile processing personnel use physical monitors to ensure that every cycle meets appropriate high-level and steam sterilization parameters by verifying printouts, digital monitors, graphs, or gauges. High-level disinfection documentation requires that designated personnel complete documentation to demonstrate compliance with local, state, and federal regulations and accrediting agency requirements, as well as ongoing documentation maintenance. ▶

Evaluate and Ensure (*continued*)

- Evaluate documentation of the following components for each reprocessed medical device: date and time of high-level disinfection processing; description of the medical device or item; medical device identification number; method of cleaning; name and title of the person performing the high-level disinfection; name of the patient on whom the device was used; name of the surgeon or physician; name of the procedure for which the medical device was used; processing exposure time; quantity of the medical devices, if appropriate to process more than one at a time; and solution temperature, lot number, expiration date, and solution test strip quality control as applicable.

- Ensure that IUSS documentation includes document cycle information and monitoring results, including cycle parameters, date and time of the cycle, items processed, monitoring results, operator information, patient identification, reason for IUSS, and type of cycle.

ALERT!

The FDA has established rules that guide manufacturers in the information they provide to health professionals on the care, treatment, use, and sterilization of materials and instruments used on patients. This information is known as Information for Use (manufacturer's recommendations).

[UNFOLDING SCENARIO 7E]

At the end of the abdominal case, the circulator wraps up documentation on the abdominal case. Part of the documentation includes logging IUSS for the Bookwalter retractor set. The nurse confirms that the date, instrument, and time are written in the log. At the end of the abdominal procedure, the scrub person is returning the instrumentation to the respective trays. The circulator notices that a blade was left on a knife handle in the tray.

Question

What other types of information should the nurse be sure to document? What should the circulator do regarding the blade left on the knife handle?

TRACKING OF MATERIALS AND INSTRUMENTS

- Tracking of materials and instruments for use in the surgical setting consists of adherence to the manufacturer's recommendations for handling and use in surgery.

- Streamlining instrument sets promotes ease of tracking and encourages the preparation of trays that have a safe weight limit, the identification of limited quantity sets, and the identification of specialty-specific instrumentation.

- This section reviews the handling of materials and instruments, IFU guidance, and regulations associated with tracking.

Assess

Assess that the perioperative nurse and the sterile processing staff are using tracking processes and facility-approved systems for instrumentation and materials according to facility policy, including instruments and devices that are new to the facility, on loan, refurbished, or repaired.

- If a facility uses a scanning system, the nurse should scan the cart as outlined in the facility's policies and procedures.

- If the facility uses a manual checking process, the nurse should adhere to the process to ensure that the contents of the cart for each case have been accounted for and to prevent delays.

Confirm

Confirm that the tracking of materials and instruments follows:

- Facility policy and AORN recommendations
- FDA standards, including approval of the instrument and device usage in surgery and review of the manufacturer's written instructions on proper cleaning and decontamination methods for the instrument and device

Evaluate and Ensure

- Evaluate surgical cases in advance and ensure that materials and instrumentation are received in the facility before the intended surgery to allow for standard terminal sterilization.

 ALERT!

TJC indicates that IUSS does not replace standard terminal sterilization and should not be used for convenience.

- Evaluate all instrumentation for ability to be powered on and off; abnormalities associated with rough edges; cleanliness; completeness; correct alignment; corrosion, pitting, burrs, and cracks; integrity of cords and insulation; and retained moisture.
- Ensure that perioperative and sterile processing personnel follow the manufacturer's IFU to avoid having to use IUSS; address the use of reprocessing for single-use devices and register with the FDA; decontaminate properly before return to the vendor; handle single-use devices; and perform sterilization processes associated with cleaning, decontaminating, high-level disinfecting, inspection, and sterilization.
- Ensure that the use of instrument and material tracking software, processes, or tools is performed according to facility policy and procedure.
- Ensure that all patient adverse events that cause harm, injury, or death are reported per facility policy and that the following FDA guidance is followed related to devices that have caused harm. The FDA can issue a tracking order for any specific device known to cause harm. Use a formal tracking mechanism for any reprocessed instrument that has been recalled.

 POP QUIZ 7.1

The circulator begins a review of the case cart for the next case using the preference list taped to the top of the cart. The facility uses a barcode scanning system for all case carts. The circulator is in a hurry and does not scan the cart. Why is this a problem?

ENVIRONMENTAL CLEANING

Environmental cleaning is the process of cleaning, disinfecting, and monitoring the environment for cleanliness. Pathogen persistence on inanimate surfaces is as follows:

- *Escherichia coli*: 1.5 hr to 16 months
- *Enterococcus faecalis*: 5 days to 4 months
- *Pseudomonas aeruginosa*: 6 hr to 16 months
- *Staphylococcus aureus*: 7 days to 7 months

Assess

Assess all areas of the surgical suite for cleanliness before opening sterile contents for the case.

Confirm

Confirm that cleaning procedures avoid the use of the following:

- Brooms with bristles to sweep the floor in semi-restricted or restricted areas
- Dry mops ▶

Confirm (*continued*)

- Items that may cause aerosolization of particulates in the air
- Self-dispensing chemical spray mops
- Spray bottles for environmental surface disinfectants

Evaluate and Ensure

Evaluate and ensure that perioperative and sterile processing personnel have cleaned high-touch areas as follows:

- Preliminary cleaning before the first case of the day: Damp dust all horizontal surfaces in OR/procedure rooms with facility-approved disinfectants.
- Interim cleaning between cases: Clean all flat surfaces and surfaces that made contact with the patient. Mop floors with damp or wet mops.
- Enhanced cleaning: Occurs when patients are infected with an MDRO or when specific pathogens (*C. difficile*, Creutzfeldt-Jakob disease [CJD], methicillin-resistant *Staphylococcus aureus* [MRSA], or tuberculosis [TB]) are present.
- Terminal cleaning in all areas daily: Clean all surfaces, including wheels and casters. Clean floors with a wet mop. Wipe down walls, ceilings, sterile storage areas, equipment rooms, ice machines, and sink.

[📝] 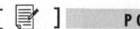 **POP QUIZ 7.2**

What should the circulator do in the surgical suite before bringing the case cart in for the next case?

ENVIRONMENTAL CONDITIONS OF THE STERILIZATION AND STORAGE AREAS

- Maintain environmental conditions and preserve the integrity of sterilized materials and instrumentation by managing humidity, temperature, moisture, and dust; heating and air ventilation systems; exposure to direct sunlight; and storage of materials and instrumentation. Limit the flow of traffic and movement around sterilized products.
- Perioperative personnel should monitor the thermostat and humidity and notify designated personnel to mitigate any issue related to heating, ventilating, and air conditioning.

Assess

Assess the surgical suite for the recommended environmental control settings as follows:

- Perioperative suite: humidity 20% to 60%; positive pressure ventilation system; temperature 68°F to 75°F (20°C–24°C)
- Sterile processing cleanroom: humidity maximum 60%; positive pressure ventilation system; temperature 68°F to 73°F (20°C–23°C)
- Endoscopy suite: humidity 20% to 60%; negative pressure for decontamination area; temperature 68°F to 73°F (20°C–23°C)
- Procedure room: humidity 20% to 60%; positive pressure ventilation system; temperature 68°F to 73°F (20°C–23°C)
- Sterile storage: humidity maximum 60%; positive pressure ventilation system; temperature maximum 75°F (24°C)

Confirm

Confirm the following is performed related to the storage of sterilized products by perioperative and sterile processing personnel: ▶

Confirm (*continued*)

- Avoid dragging wrapped material to prevent tearing of wrapping.
- Use dust covers when appropriate.
- Follow hand hygiene and surgical attire practices per facility policies.
- Ensure shelving is free from damage or burrs that could damage packaging.
- Configure shelving and space to ensure adequate air circulation from all angles.
- Ensure that stacking occurs per the manufacturer's IFU.

Evaluate and Ensure

- Evaluate and ensure that traffic and movement are limited in relation to stored sterilized materials and instrumentation.
- Ensure CDC and AORN guidelines are followed related to the storage of sterile materials and instrumentation. Date every sterilized product; monitor sterility of all sterile products on a routine basis; store sterile supplies and instruments in areas free from moisture, such as in closed cabinets or covered racks; store sterile supplies 8 to 10 in. from the floor, 5 in. from the ceiling, 18 in. from a sprinkler head, and 2 in. from an outside wall; and use the facility-approved shelf-life practice for evaluating sterile materials (e.g., event related or time related).

HANDLING OF HAZARDOUS AND BIOHAZARDOUS MATERIALS

The perioperative nurse works to reduce risks associated with selecting, transporting, handling, and disposing of hazardous materials. Hazardous materials include those that cause radiation exposure, chemical exposure, or blood-borne pathogen exposure.

Assess

- Assess the risks associated with handling hazardous and biohazardous materials for each case.
- Assess the surgical suite for the presence of adequate PPE supply, correct distance from the surgical suite to the nearest eyewash station and scrub sink, and supplies to confine and contain biohazardous fluid spills.

Confirm

- Confirm that all perioperative personnel and visitors work to minimize radiation exposure by maintaining a distance of 6 ft. from the radiation source, remaining behind leaded shielding when ionizing radiation use occurs, protecting the patient with appropriate lead shielding, and wearing protective lead and moving as far as possible away from the source while maintaining aseptic technique for scrubbed personnel.
- Confirm that perioperative personnel report biohazardous exposures (blood, bodily fluids, chemicals, and radiation) to the employer per OSHA guidelines.

Evaluate and Ensure

- Evaluate the need for the following protective equipment and ensure its use by all personnel and when appropriate for the patient within the surgical suite when radiation exposure is likely: flexible leaded aprons; lead vests, skirts, thyroid shields, and gloves; leaded safety eyeglasses with side shields; PPE for radioactive chemicals and drugs; and rigid shields on wheels. ▶

[ ]   **ALERT!**

When managing a case associated with CJD, which is a fatal neurodegenerative disease:

- Use disposable instrumentation sets for diagnostic brain biopsies to rule out CJD or transmissible spongiform encephalopathy (TSE).
- Do not use chemical or physical methods, including steam autoclaving, dry heat, or ethylene oxide gas. Chemical disinfection with formaldehyde or glutaraldehyde will destroy the prions that cause the disease.

Evaluate and Ensure (*continued*)

- Ensure that all members of the perioperative team don the appropriate PPE to protect against blood-borne pathogen transmission through the following: debris—tissue or blood on instrumentation, sharps, and needlesticks; fluids—cerebrospinal fluid, synovial fluid, pleural fluid, peritoneal fluid, and amniotic fluid; secretions—semen, vaginal discharge, saliva, and mucus; tissue—central nervous system tissue.
- Ensure hand hygiene is performed after the following occurs: patient contact, removal of gloves, touching blood or body fluids, and touching contaminated items.
- Ensure compliance with OSHA blood-borne pathogen standards relating to reducing exposure to blood, bodily fluids, and infectious or hazardous materials. Attend training on the prevention of occupational exposure to blood, bodily fluids, and hazardous chemicals. Restrict the activities of personnel who have infections, open lesions, or nonintact skin. Use safety devices, neutral zones, and hands-free techniques to reduce exposure to sharps injuries. Wear PPE at all times.
- Ensure that infectious and noninfectious tissues and waste are managed according to OSHA and AORN's position statement for environmental responsibility. Eliminate mercury-based products. Follow the waste removal protocols established by the organization related to recycling, disposal, dilution, or deactivation (e.g., radioactive or other chemical fluids). Limit the use of biohazardous waste containers to infectious waste (e.g., red bag). Survey the type of waste that is projected to be produced by the procedure and plan availability of requisite equipment and supplies for potential spillage and collection. Use a bag-in-bag collection system to reduce the risks to healthcare workers.

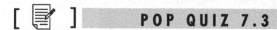

POP QUIZ 7.3

The circulating nurse is preparing for a patient scheduled to undergo an open reduction internal fixation of the left ankle. The nurse opens a tray of instruments and discovers moisture. What is the appropriate next step?

RESOURCES

Association of periOperative Registered Nurses. (2019). *Guideline essentials: Key takeaways. Sterilization.* https://www.aorn.org/essentials/sterilization

Association of periOperative Registered Nurses. (2020a). AORN position statement on environmental responsibility. *AORN Journal, 111*(6), 1–11. https://doi.org/10.1002/aorn.13063

Association of periOperative Registered Nurses. (2020b). *Guideline essentials: Key takeaways. Environmental cleaning.* https://www.aorn.org/essentials/environmental-cleaning

Association of periOperative Registered Nurses. (2020c). *Guideline essentials: Key takeaways. Packaging.* https://www.aorn.org/essentials/packaging-systems

Association of periOperative Registered Nurses. (2021a). *Guideline for design and maintenance, guidelines for perioperative practice.* Author.

Association of periOperative Registered Nurses. (2021b). *Guideline for environmental cleaning, guidelines for perioperative practice.* Author.

Association of periOperative Registered Nurses. (2021c). *Guideline for environment of care, guidelines for perioperative practice.* Author.

Association of periOperative Registered Nurses. (2021d). *Guideline for hand hygiene, guidelines for perioperative practice.* Author.

Association of periOperative Registered Nurses. (2021e). *Guideline for high level disinfection, guidelines for perioperative practice.* Author.

Association of periOperative Registered Nurses. (2021f). *Guideline for instrument cleaning, guidelines for perioperative practice.* Author.

Association of periOperative Registered Nurses. (2021g). *Guideline for packaging systems, guidelines for perioperative practice*. Author.

Association of periOperative Registered Nurses. (2021h). *Guideline for radiation safety, guidelines for perioperative practice*. Author.

Association of periOperative Registered Nurses. (2021i). *Guideline for sharps safety, guidelines for perioperative practice*. Author.

Association of periOperative Registered Nurses. (2021j). *Guideline for sterile technique, guidelines for perioperative practice*. Author.

Association of periOperative Registered Nurses. (2021k). *Guideline for sterilization, guidelines for perioperative practice*. Author.

Association of periOperative Registered Nurses. (2021l). *Guideline for surgical attire, guidelines for perioperative practice*. Author.

Berríos-Torres, S. I., Umscheid, C. A., Bratzler, D. W., Leas, B., Stone, E. C., Kelz, R. R., Reinke, C. E., Morgan, S., Solomkin, J. S., Mazuski, J. E., Dellinger, E. P., Itani, K. M. F., Berbari, E. F., Segreti, J., Parvizi, J., Blanchard, J., Allen, G., Kluytmans, J. A. J. W., Donlan, R., & Schecter, W. P. (2017). Centers for Disease Control and Prevention guideline for the prevention of surgical site infection, 2017. *JAMA Surgery, 152*(8), 784–791. https://doi.org/10.1001/jamasurg.2017.0904

Centers for Disease Control and Prevention. (n.d.-a). *Standard precautions for all patient care*. U.S. Department of Health and Human Services, Centers for Disease Control and Prevention. https://www.cdc.gov/infection control/basics/standard-precautions.html

Centers for Disease Control and Prevention. (n.d.-b). *Transmission-based precautions*. U.S. Department of Health and Human Services, Centers for Disease Control and Prevention. https://www.cdc.gov/infectioncontrol/basics/transmission-based-precautions.html

The Joint Commission. (2013). *The Joint Commission's implementation guide for NPSG.07.05.01 on surgical site infections: The SSI change project*. https://www.jointcommission.org/-/media/tjc/documents/resources/hai/implementation_guide_for_npsg_ssipdf.pdf

The Joint Commission. (2021a, January 1). *Hospital: 2021 national patient safety goals*. https://www.joint commission.org/standards/national-patient-safety-goals/hospital-national-patient-safety-goals

The Joint Commission. (2021b, March 1). *Instrument reprocessing—Immediate use steam sterilization (IUSS): What are important considerations associated with immediate-use steam sterilization?* https://www.jointcommission.org/standards/standard-faqs/ambulatory/infection-prevention-and-control-ic/000002122

The Joint Commission. (n.d). *Surgical site infections*. https://www.jointcommission.org/resources/patient-safety-topics/infection-prevention-and-control/surgical-site-infections

Occupational Safety and Health Administration. (n.d.-a). *Bloodborne pathogens and needlestick prevention*. United States Department of Labor, Occupational Safety and Health Administration. https://www.osha.gov/blood borne-pathogens/standards

Occupational Safety and Health Administration. (n.d.-b). *Personal protective equipment*. United States Department of Labor, Occupational Safety and Health Administration. https://www.osha.gov/personal-protective-equipment

Rothrock, J. C. (Ed.). (2019). *Alexander's care of the patient in surgery* (16th ed.). Elsevier—Health Sciences Division.

EMERGENCY SITUATIONS

OVERVIEW

- Emergency situations can arise at any time in the perioperative suite. This chapter reviews some of the most common emergent situations, including anaphylaxis; conversion to an open procedure; difficult airway; environmental hazards; hemorrhage; local anesthetic systemic toxicity (LAST); malignant hyperthermia (MH); mass casualty, triage, and evacuation; perioperative cardiac arrest; and trauma.
- Throughout each phase of the perioperative experience, the nurse will perform duties using the ACE process: **A**ssess, **C**onfirm, and **E**valuate and **E**nsure.

ANAPHYLAXIS

Anaphylaxis is a type I hypersensitivity reaction and medical emergency that occurs in response to exposure to an allergen. The occurrence of anaphylaxis in the OR is rare. It is primarily related to latex exposure associated with products used for patient handling and the procedure, neuromuscular blocking drugs, or antibiotic allergies that are unknown to the patient.

Assess

- Assess the patient and family history for allergic reactions to the following: antibiotics, induction medications, intraoperative medications and fluorescent dyes (hyaluronidase, methylene blue, coagulation agents, trypan blue, indocyanine green, and colloids), latex, neuromuscular blocking drugs, and skin prepping agents (chlorhexidine, betadine, and alcohol).
- Assess the patient for risk factors associated with latex sensitivity, such as food allergies (banana, kiwi, avocado, chestnut, and raw potato), history of long-term bladder care, spina bifida, spinal cord trauma, urogenital abnormalities, or multiple procedures, and symptoms associated with asthma, dermatitis, urticaria, hay fever, or rhinitis.
- Assess the patient for signs and symptoms of anaphylactic reactions. Table 8.1 lists common signs and symptoms.
- Assess the patient's skin postoperatively for signs and symptoms of dermatitis, erythema, edema, or impaired skin integrity.

> **[⚙] ALERT!**
>
> For patients with known latex allergy, remove all items that might contain latex, such as gloves, catheters, intravenous line (IV) equipment, tape, tourniquets, ventilation and airway equipment, and medication stoppers.

Confirm

Confirm the following:

- All drugs used during the procedure are verified with the surgeon and anesthesia personnel before dispensing to the field.
- Epinephrine is available and ready for use on the patient during the emergency. ▶

TABLE 8.1	Signs and Symptoms of Anaphylactic Reactions
BODY SYSTEM	**SIGNS AND SYMPTOMS**
Cardiovascular	Tachycardia, hypotension, arrhythmias
Genitourinary	Reduced urine output
Hematologic	DIC
Integumentary	Urticaria, pruritis, edema, erythema
Respiratory	Dyspnea, hypoxia, pulmonary edema, bronchospasm, increased respirations

DIC, disseminated intravascular coagulation.

Confirm (*continued*)

- Patient-reported allergies are shared with all members of the surgical team.
- The causative agent and associated products are discontinued and removed rapidly upon patient presentation with anaphylaxis.

Evaluate and Ensure

- Ensure the following have been completed intraoperatively and in preparation for an anaphylactic reaction: confirmation that medications that will serve to counteract the reaction (epinephrine, vasopressin, diphenhydramine, ranitidine, famotidine, hydrocortisone, methylprednisolone, and albuterol) are available; confirmation that low-protein and powder-free gloves are available; latex precautions for patients with known latex sensitivity or allergy; presence of the code cart and defibrillator in the surgical suite; protection of the sterile field by the scrub person during the emergency; restriction of traffic in the surgical suite; and placement of signs and patient armbands for patients who have a latex or medication allergy.
- Evaluate the code cart to ensure that the contents have been checked according to facility policy and the defibrillator is operational.

CONVERSION TO AN OPEN PROCEDURE

- Conversion to an open procedure can occur with laparoscopic and robotic surgical approaches. ▶

 NURSING PEARL

Use the **ALLERGIC** mnemonic to remember how to proactively protect the patient from an allergic reaction:

- **A**ssess the patient for known allergies.
- **L**atex products must be removed if a problem.
- **L**imit the traffic in the suite.
- **E**pinephrine bolus and fluids should be available.
- **R**escue drugs and code cart should be available.
- **G**love selection should be appropriate based on patient allergies.
- **I**solate and protect the sterile field.
- **C**ausative agents should be identified.

 POP QUIZ 8.1

A 42-year-old nulliparous female presents to the OR for a bilateral breast mastectomy related to the finding of breast cancer in both breasts. She has a medical history of hypertension and diabetes mellitus (DM). Both conditions are well controlled. During the preoperative assessment, the patient reports having an allergic reaction to penicillin, which causes a rash. This is the patient's first surgical procedure. The surgeon indicates that she will also perform sentinel node biopsy and lymphatic mapping and asks that isosulfan blue dye be dispensed to the surgical field. The patient will be administered general anesthesia.

During the procedure, the surgeon begins the lymphatic mapping and injects the isosulfan blue dye. The anesthesiologist alerts the surgeon that the patient's blood pressure has dropped to 62/40 and her heart rate has spiked to 125 bpm. The patient also exhibits labored breathing. What is happening to the patient, and what should the circulating nurse do next?

CONVERSION TO AN OPEN PROCEDURE (*CONTINUED*)

- Conversion is considered an emergent situation and will occur when complications arise, including the following: bleeding or hemorrhage from a puncture, tissue cuts and tears, suture or surgical clip failure, or other vessel disruption; gas embolism, which can cause cardiovascular collapse; hypothermia from carbon dioxide insufflation colder than the body temperature of the patient; incidental iatrogenic injury from positioning aids, port placement, surgical errors, robotic attachments, or placement of other equipment; perforation of a major organ or vessel related to trocars and rigid scopes used during surgery; and preperitoneal insufflation from gas that has not been evacuated using the inlet side port, which occurs when a trocar instead of a Veress needle is used to insufflate.

[ ] **NURSING PEARL**

Use the **CONVERT** mnemonic when converting to an open procedure from a laparoscopic procedure and when the risk of hemorrhage is evident:

- **C**all for help.
- **O**pen additional supplies as needed.
- **N**otify the blood bank.
- **V**erify blood products.
- **E**mergency code cart should be obtained.
- **R**emove all contents from the surgical wound and perform a count when feasible.
- **T**urn all lights on and turn off the fiber optic light source to prevent fire.

Assess

- Assess for potential anesthesia factors that could contribute to conversion to an open procedure from either laparoscopic or robotic surgical procedure, such as inadequate muscle relaxation for the procedure, ineffective hemodynamic stability, and respiratory instability associated with insufflation and hypoxia.

- Assess for surgical factors that can contribute to conversion to an open procedure from either a laparoscopic or robotic surgical procedure, such as hemorrhage related to surgical error or change in patient's status, manipulation of the robot master controls, placement of ports, skill set related to the use of the robotic system or laparoscopic trocars and instruments, and testing of systems related to laparoscopic or robotic procedures (insufflation, electrocautery unit, foot pedals and connections, video tower and power sources, etc.).

- Assess for potential technical factors that can contribute to conversion to an open procedure from either a laparoscopic or robotic surgical procedure, such as, technical issues related to equipment or instrumentation, and video imaging issues that cause insufficient visibility.

- Assess the consent and ensure that the potential to convert to an open procedure is written on the consent.

[ ] **POP QUIZ 8.2**

A 62-year-old patient presents to the OR suite for laparoscopic cholecystectomy. The patient is positioned, intubated, draped, and prepped. The time-out is performed. The surgical incision has been made, and the first port is placed using the Hassan technique. Insufflation of the abdominal cavity has commenced. The surgeon introduces the laparoscope with the RN first assistant (RNFA) standing by to place the next port. When the surgeon advances the laparoscope, it shows multiple adhesions wrapped around the liver and adjacent organs. The surgeon notes that the gallbladder is oozing due to pressure from the adhesions. The surgeon alerts the anesthesiologist that the case will need to convert to an open procedure. The anesthesiologist begins to stabilize the patient for the change in position. The surgeon begins to decompress the abdomen and release the gas. What is the role of the circulating nurse in this scenario?

Confirm

- Confirm that the following have been performed related to conversion to an open procedure from the robotic or laparoscopic procedure: Complete a full count of all instrumentation, sharps, and sponges at the beginning of the procedure in preparation for potential conversion; follow facility policy on the need to perform a second time-out for robotic procedures during which each member of the team verbalizes what should be done in the event of conversion to an open procedure; notify or page additional surgeons as requested by the attending surgeon; open additional instrumentation, sharps, and sponges as needed; safely disconnect all cords attached to the equipment for lights, ultrasonic, and other power sources that will not be used during the open procedure; turn on the overhead lights and or lights; and undock the robot.

Evaluate and Ensure

- Evaluate the type of emergency associated with the procedure (technical, surgical, or anesthetic).
- Evaluate the patient assessment performed by the surgeon and confer with the surgical team on the reasons conversion to an open procedure might occur, such as distorted anatomy that would inhibit safe dissection, gross contamination or infection within a cavity, hemorrhage, patient's intolerance to pneumoperitoneum or the required positioning or concerns raised by the anesthesia personnel related to the inability to provide safe respiratory support, and the presence of abdominal adhesions.
- Ensure that the patient is prepped and draped in a manner that will preserve sterility at the field and in preparation for potential conversion to an open procedure.
- Ensure that the time of conversion and any changes in patient status are recorded in the nursing documentation.

DIFFICULT AIRWAY

There are times when a patient presents to the OR suite with a difficult airway related to a medical emergency, the patient's medical and surgical history, or congenital or acquired anatomic defects of the airway.

The presentation of a difficult airway is often unanticipated and creates challenges for the anesthesia team related to airway management. Although the management of the patient's airway falls under the scope of practice for anesthesia personnel, the perioperative nurse must provide support to the patient and the anesthesia team by being present at the bedside during induction and emergence.

[ ]   **NURSING PEARL**

The American Society of Anesthesiology (ASA) defines a *difficult airway* as a "clinical situation wherein a trained anesthesiologist cannot achieve effective facemask ventilation of the upper airway, establish tracheal intubation, or both."

Assess

- Assess the patient's medical history associated with congenital or acquired anatomic defects; history of facial, neck, or chest trauma; and history of regurgitation, obesity, or oral cavity disease.

Confirm

- Confirm availability of the airway management supplies.
- Confirm that the patient is in the appropriate position to maximize exposure for intubation.

Evaluate and Ensure

- Evaluate the patient's response to activities occurring within the sterile field throughout the entire procedure.
- Ensure the following associated with patient safety: Patient is positioned so that the head is in neutral alignment with the vertebral axis, the cervical spine is stable, and the head is slightly extended. Support is provided to the anesthesia team by remaining at the head of the bed and providing necessary assistance related to the application of cricoid pressure, inflation of the cuff, or removal of the stylet. The safety strap is securely placed in an area that maximizes exposure to the surgical site and does not constrict breathing.

POP QUIZ 8.3

A 65-year-old man presents to the OR suite directly from the emergency room with a possible ruptured appendix. The report from the emergency room physician indicates that the patient said he had been vomiting, has had diarrhea for over 24 hr, and is experiencing intense pain in the right lower abdomen. During induction, the anesthesiologist reports that intubation through direct laryngoscopy is difficult. The nurse anesthetist retrieves the difficult airway cart. What is the role of the perioperative circulating nurse?

ENVIRONMENTAL HAZARD EMERGENCIES

- The perioperative nurse must work with the surgical team to mitigate the risks associated with environmental hazards in and around the surgical suite. Environmental hazards in the surgical suite include the following: blood-borne pathogens and hazardous waste; chemical exposure; compressed gases; communicable disease exposure; equipment burns or shocks; fire; laser use; radiation exposure; slips, trips, and falls; smoke plume; and waste anesthetic gases.

Assess

Assess the surgical suite continuously for potential environmental hazards.

Confirm

The perioperative nurse should confirm with the surgical team that the potential for occupational injury from exposure to harmful chemicals, waste, and pathogens has been evaluated and voice any concerns before the start of a procedure.

Evaluate and Ensure

Evaluate for and ensure that actions are taken to mitigate injury associated with environmental hazards. Table 8.2 lists common environmental hazards and associated nursing actions.

NURSING PEARL

Working to prevent injury in the work environment is essential. Benjamin Franklin once said, "An ounce of prevention is worth a pound of cure."

POP QUIZ 8.4

The OR suite has been prepped for a right shoulder arthroscopy with rotator cuff repair. As the procedure commences, the perioperative circulating nurse performs a safety evaluation. The nurse notes that multiple cords and equipment affect the traffic pattern in the surgical suite. What is the best course of action for the nurse to take to ensure safety?

HEMORRHAGE

- With surgical intervention comes the risk of blood loss associated with hemorrhage due to medical error or anatomic dysfunction. Disseminated intravascular coagulation (DIC) is associated with hemorrhage and is also a complication in surgery. *DIC* is an acquired systemic disorder that involves a combination of hemorrhage and microvascular coagulation. Hemorrhage and DIC are unexpected medical emergencies that can occur in the OR.

TABLE 8.2	Environmental Hazards and Actions
HAZARDS	**ACTIONS**
Blood-borne pathogens and hazardous waste	• Routinely replace all sharps containers to ensure there is a means for disposing of sharps safely. • Ensure all staff are wearing appropriate PPE in anticipation of exposure to blood-borne pathogens, chemicals, and laser use. • Promote the use of double-gloving, blunted needles, and safe zones for the passing of sharps.
Chemical exposure	• Handle and store all chemicals according to the manufacturer's recommendation and MSDS (disinfectants, sterilants, tissue preservatives, antiseptic agents). • Educate staff on the use of eyewash stations based on facility policy. • Ensure eyewash stations are plumbed or self-contained and in close proximity to where chemicals are handled. • Review emergency spill plans and respiratory protection plans with staff and keep copies in an area in close proximity to where chemicals are handled.
Communicable disease exposure	• Follow facility, state, local, and federal guidelines associated with identification, isolation, and treatment of patients with communicable diseases (TB, HIV/AIDS, etc.). • Maintain PPE protocols associated with the organism. • Maintain the appropriate air exchanges associated with caring for a patient with a communicable disease. • Reduce airborne particle spread by restricting traffic within the suite.
Compressed gases	• Check cylinders before use for evidence of the appropriate labeling, color-coding, and pin safety according to facility policy. • Store an emergency supply of oxygen according to facility policy. • Store medical gases in a secured location away from industrial gases and routes of egress. • Transport medical gases in facility-approved carriers that are designed to prevent cylinders from being dropped or tipped. • Use approved fittings, flow control devices, and regulators associated with the medical gas.
Equipment burns or shocks	• Inspect all electrical equipment for damage and integrity of the cord insulation. • Remove equipment with frayed cords or damage and report per facility procedure. • Use devices according to manufacturers' guidelines.
Fire	• Perform a fire safety assessment before each case associated with ignition sources, fuels, and the potential for an oxygen-enriched environment. • Prevent contact between fuels (e.g., alcohol-based skin antiseptic agents, drapes, and gowns) and ignition sources. • Use ignition sources according to manufacturer's guidelines (e.g., electrosurgical electrodes, fiber-optic light cords).
Laser use	• Attach extra laser protective eyewear to the door with a sign. • Cover windows in the nominal hazard zone with a barrier that blocks the laser beam. • Display warning signs on each door of the surgical suite. • Ensure that the laser has been maintained and checked by facility-authorized technicians. • Limit the traffic in the suite to those who are trained in laser safety precautions. • Perform appropriate calibration of the beam before each procedure. • Perform a laser-safety time-out before the start of the laser procedure. • Place laser in standby mode when not in use. • Use appropriate filters or barriers according to OSHA standards. • Use laser protective eyewear.

(continued)

TABLE 8.2 Environmental Hazards and Actions (*continued*)	
HAZARDS	**ACTIONS**
Radiation exposure	• Protect the patient from radiation exposure by applying the appropriate lead shield after the patient has been positioned for surgery. • Wear a passive dosimeter to monitor personal radiation exposure associated with x-ray equipment and radioactive patients or materials. • Wear appropriate lead aprons, gloves, thyroid shields, and goggles when in contact with radiation.
Slips, trips, and falls	• Arrange equipment and supplies so that the suite is not cluttered, and pathways are not obstructed. • Cover electrical cables on the floor with a facility-approved cord cover. • Provide appropriate lighting within the suite. • Post signs where wet floor hazards exist. • Rapidly clean up spills or debris. • Wear slip-resistant shoes or facility-approved shoe covers.
Smoke plume	• Treat all tubing, filters, and absorbers as infectious waste. • Routinely inspect smoke evacuation equipment for proper functioning. • Use smoke evacuation equipment and inline suction filters for each case.
Waste anesthetic gases	• Provide enough ventilation to keep the room concentration of waste anesthetic gases below occupational exposure levels. • Report issues with ventilation and air exchanges promptly to the manager.

MSDS, material safety data sheets; PPE, personalized protective equipment; TB, tuberculosis.

Assess

■ Assess laboratory test data for prolonged bleeding times (e.g., prothrombin time [PT], activated partial thromboplastin time [aPPT], and international normalized ratio [INR] values).
■ Assess the patient's medical and surgical history for previous issues with tissue healing.

Confirm

■ Confirm that the patient has had a blood type, cross, and screen in preparation for planned blood loss during the procedure.
■ Confirm availability of blood products with the laboratory.

Evaluate and Ensure

■ Evaluate for signs and symptoms of DIC (e.g., profuse bleeding at the surgical site, petechiae).
■ Ensure the following are addressed related to blood transfusion: A two-person confirmation of blood products and patient identification is performed. Blood products are handled safely, and standard PPE is used. Blood products are used within the time frame indicated by the facility and in accordance with the American Association of Blood Blanks guidelines. Transfusion reactions are noted in the perioperative record. ▶

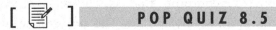

POP QUIZ 8.5

A 47-year-old male is undergoing a laparoscopic cholecystectomy that requires emergent conversion to open procedure because the cystic artery is cut. The surgeon states that the patient is hemorrhaging. What should the circulating nurse do to assist in this situation?

Evaluate and Ensure (*continued*)

■ Ensure the following are addressed related to emergencies associated with perioperative hemorrhage: Off the field, dispense medications and other medical supplies as ordered by the surgeon in a timely fashion. Provide support to anesthesia personnel related to the acquisition of blood products as needed. On the field, remove all sharps and other surgical products from the surgical field and account for all while the surgeon works to find the source of the bleeding.

LOCAL ANESTHETIC SYSTEMIC TOXICITY

■ *LAST* is a life-threatening adverse event that involves the central nervous system (CNS) and may be caused by the rate of absorption at the injection site, the injection technique, the type of anesthetic used, and/or patient characteristics.

Assess

■ Assess patient characteristics that may increase the risk of LAST, such as disease processes associated with the liver, heart, pregnancy, and metabolic syndromes; extremes of age; known cardiac conduction or electrolyte abnormality; and low body mass index (BMI).

Confirm

Confirm the dosage and route of the local injection with the surgeon.

Evaluate and Ensure

■ Evaluate the patient for the following from 30 seconds to 60 minutes following injection: Use EKG monitoring for asystole, bradycardia, ventricular fibrillation, and wide-QRS complex ventricular tachycardia. Symptoms include confusion or disorientation, dizziness, drowsiness, local tissue response, metallic taste, and oral numbness.

■ Ensure the following are completed if LAST is suspected: Assist with administration of 20% lipid emulsion therapy, assist with resuscitation, call for help (code team, anesthesia personnel), establish or assist with IV access, maintain the airway, stop the administration of the local anesthetic, and ventilate with 100% oxygen.

MALIGNANT HYPERTHERMIA

Malignant hyperthermia (MH) is an inherited pharmacogenetic syndrome that is caused by anesthetic agents and succinylcholine. The occurrence of MH in the operating suite is a life-threatening adverse event requiring swift action of the entire perioperative team to avert the progression of the crisis and patient death. The anesthesia team will alert the surgeon that an MH crisis is apparent, at which time the surgical procedure will come to a halt and life-saving measures will ensue.

 NURSING PEARL

The LAST rescue kit should include a lipid emulsion 20%, large syringes (50 mL), IV administration supplies, and the American Society of Regional Anesthesia checklist. See the Resources section for list details.

 POP QUIZ 8.6

A 61-year-old male is admitted to the perioperative suite for an excision of a lipoma on the right leg. He has a low BMI and atrial fibrillation. His past surgical history includes a bilateral inguinal hernia repair and a laparoscopic appendectomy. He reports having no adverse effects to anesthesia during past surgeries. At the start of the procedure, the surgeon requests that 0.5% bupivacaine and 1% lidocaine be dispensed to the sterile field for local injection. The surgeon injects 10 mL of lidocaine combined with 2 mL of bupivacaine at the start of the procedure. Five minutes after the injection, the patient displays confusion, says that his mouth feels numb, and becomes bradycardic. What should the circulating nurse do in response to the change in the patient's condition?

Assess

Assess the patient's medical record related to the following:

- Allergies to medications or foods
- Anxiety and pain level
- Assistive devices
- Current medications
- Implanted devices
- Medical and surgical history
- Previous anesthesia complications

Confirm

- In known cases of complications associated with anesthesia, the nurse should confirm that the triggering agents are removed from the anesthesia workstation.
- The nurse should also confirm that the anesthetic agent has been properly flushed from the system and that all delivery lines and suction are new.
- The nurse should confirm that the MH cart is available.

Evaluate and Ensure

- Evaluate for any changes in the patient's status throughout the procedure.
- Ensure the following activities are completed during an MH crisis to assist anesthesia personnel: Stop the use of volatile agents and succinylcholine. Retrieve the following pharmacologic treatment products— two 10-mL vials of calcium chloride (10%); 2.5 mg/kg of antrolene sodium; 50-mL vials of dextrose 50%; three 100 mg/5 mL or 100 mg/10 mL of lidocaine for injection (2%) in preloaded syringes; 100 units/mL of regular insulin, refrigerated; a minimum of 3,000 mL of refrigerated saline for IV cooling; five 50-mL vials

of sodium bicarbonate (8.4%); sterile water for injection USP (United States Pharmacopeia; without a bacteriostatic agent) to reconstitute dantrolene. Retrieve the following nonpharmacologic treatments— ice lavage through the esophagus or rectal tube, and ice packs around the patient's body, head, and feet. Retrieve equipment/supplies that may be used during an MH crisis—activated charcoal filters; blood gas kits; central venous pressure kits (sizes appropriate to patient population); crushed ice and plastic bags; esophageal and other core temperature probes; syringes, needles, and transfer devices; transducer kits for arterial and central venous cannulation; and urimeter. Report the crisis to the management team, Malignant Hyperthermia Association of the United States (MHAUS), and the post-anesthesia care unit (PACU) or ICU. Report to MHAUS by calling the MHAUS Hotline (1-800-644-9737 or outside the United States 001-209-417-3722) for additional advice. A trained MH anesthesia person will join the anesthesiologist of record for the case to help to guide the crisis.

NURSING PEARL

STOP what you are doing in an MH crisis:

- Stop the volatile agents and succinylcholine.
- Treat the patient with supportive care, dantrolene, and cooling.
- *Oxygen 100%:* Use to flush out the volatile anesthetics.
- Prepare to cool the patient with ice and IV saline.

POP QUIZ 8.7

A healthy 17-year-old male is positioned for a right inguinal hernia repair. The patient has no prior surgical history. His parents report he has not had complications with anesthetic agents. Fifteen minutes into the surgery, the patient begins to exhibit signs and symptoms such as buccal rigidity, rapid heart rate, and decreased oxygen saturation rate. The anesthesiologist alerts the surgeon that the patient is experiencing MH. The surgeon stops the procedure and begins to close the wound. What should the perioperative circulating nurse initially do to assist the team?

MASS CASUALTY, TRIAGE, AND EVACUATION

- The perioperative nurse must be prepared to manage casualties caused by human-made and natural disasters.
- The facility policy for the management of casualty events and evacuation from the facility should be reviewed regularly to ensure that all staff are aware of the steps to take to triage patients, manage care, and prepare the OR to receive patients in an expedited manner.

Assess

- Assess the mass casualty event policy and plan to coordinate with the interprofessional team as well as outside agencies to coordinate patient care.
- Assess the population of patients and the resources needed to safely evacuate patients if a mass casualty event occurs in the healthcare facility.
- Assess the type of exposure or injuries expected (e.g., chemical, biologic, radiologic, nuclear, or incendiary incidents).

Confirm

- Confirm the following associated with the evacuation of patients: assembly of the patients according to ambulatory status, nonambulatory status, wheelchair-bound, mobility deficit, and critical care needs when moving patients who have critical care needs.
- Confirm the following associated with triaging patients: availability of resources needed for incoming cases and use of the facility-approved system for prioritization of patients.

Evaluate and Ensure

- Evaluate the supply lists generated for incoming cases and alert management if there will be any challenges or barriers related to the availability of products.
- Ensure that patients' needs are addressed in a timely fashion related to the level of triage, according to facility policy and AORN guidelines. Critical or emergent ranking requires surgical treatment of patients immediately, whereas semi-critical requires surgical intervention within 6 to 8 hr.
- Ensure that the goals associated with surgical intervention in a mass casualty event are met, including the following: appropriate space available to assess and triage patients; availability of blood and blood products; availability of necessary equipment, instrumentation, and other medical supplies; documentation of all interventions and barriers to providing care; identification of team members who are skilled and trained to perform; reduction in delays through efficient use of resources and time; saving the most lives; and use of AORN standards and facility policy.
- Ensure the following are addressed related to facility-wide evacuation: documentation of all patients and personnel evacuated; effective communication between facilities and team personnel; identification of patient's needs during the transfer of care; mode of transportation; preparation of patient's medical records and medications; and routes of egress and types of evacuation.

[📝] **POP QUIZ 8.8**

The OR department manager is notified that there is an electrical fire in the building adjacent to the OR and a code red is in effect. The facilities director tells the OR manager that all procedures are to be halted where feasible and evacuation orders are received. The patients must be evacuated to the first floor of the hospital. The OR is on the third floor. The cases running are as follows:

- A cystoscopy in mid-procedure
- A laparoscopic cholecystectomy case wrapping up
- A total hip arthroplasty that just started
- A tracheostomy for an ICU patient that just started
- Four patients in the holding area
- One patient on the way to the OR suite to undergo a total knee arthroplasty

What type of evacuation would be used in this scenario, and who might the nurse prepare to move first?

PERIOPERATIVE CARDIAC ARREST

During the intraoperative and postoperative period, the patient undergoes substantial physiologic stress. The once-stable patient may decompensate intraoperatively or during the postoperative period, which could lead to complications such as nonfatal myocardial infarction, pulmonary edema, ventricular tachycardia, or patient death.

Assess

Assess the patient for risks associated with cardiac arrest:

- Age (men older than 45 years and women older than 55 years)
- History of myocardial infarction, stroke, coronary artery disease (CAD), cardiomyopathy, or heart disease
- Obesity or sedentary lifestyle
- Social habits (e.g., smoking, alcohol abuse, illicit drug use)

Confirm

Confirm the presence of the emergency code cart during a cardiac arrest situation.

Evaluate and Ensure

- Evaluate the situation and call for the emergency code cart.
- Ensure the following assistive actions are provided to the anesthesia team and surgeon during a perioperative cardiac arrest: Document all aspects of the process associated with cardiac life support, facilitate the protection of the sterile table by limiting traffic and movement, and provide assistance with cardiopulmonary resuscitation as directed by the anesthesiologist and/or surgeon.

[ ]   **NURSING PEARL**

The steps of the cardiac event process include the following:

- Retrieve the emergency code cart.
- Assist with repositioning the patient.
- Perform chest compressions as needed.
- Notify the OR manager.
- Inform the code leader of tasks performed.
- Maintain sterility of the field and surgical counts.
- Control the traffic in the room.
- Document all interventions.

[ ]   **POP QUIZ 8.9**

An 80-year-old woman presents to the OR for a cervical discectomy and is placed in the prone position. The patient has hypertension and a history of myocardial infarction that occurred 5 years ago. The patient is anesthetized, positioned, prepped, and draped. Twenty minutes after the surgical incision is made, the patient develops ventricular tachycardia followed by ventricular fibrillation and cardiac arrest. What should the circulating nurse do first to assist the team in managing the issue?

TRAUMA

- Trauma is associated with blunt force and penetrating injuries. Traumatic injuries affect internal organs, bones, the brain, and other soft tissue. These types of injuries are treated as medical emergencies that may cause direct admission into the OR from the emergency department. They may be caused by catastrophic falls, crushing injuries, motor vehicle accidents, stabbings, or gunshot wounds.
- All perioperative nursing care of the trauma patient is contoured to meet needs associated with the nature of the injury. Equipment, instruments, other medical supplies, and positioning requirements are based on surgeon preference and the needs for the particular case.

Assess

- Assess the patient's history, physical and laboratory data and related documentation, and physical presentation. ▶

Assess (*continued*)

- Assess the family's presence and coping mechanisms related to the patient's condition.
- Assess for signs of bleeding.
- Assess according to the following nursing diagnoses related to trauma: acute pain, anxiety and fear, deficient fluid volume, risk for aspiration, and risk for hypothermia.
- Obtain as much information as possible if the patient is awake, alert, and oriented.
- Assess the patient using the **ABCDE** primary survey method (Rothrock, 2019): **A**irway assessment, **B**reathing and ventilation status, **C**irculation assessment and hemorrhage status, **D**isability related to neurologic issues, and **E**xposure to injury requiring a full head-to-toe assessment.
- Assess the patient related to the type of trauma: Blunt trauma results from automobile accidents or assaults and may be caused by an airbag being deployed, contact with the steering wheel, direction of the impact and distance associated with ejection from a vehicle, and seat belt restraint. Penetrating trauma results from gunshot wounds or stabbing and is characterized by distance from the firearm and the point of contact, length of the blade, number of wounds, and type of the firearm, blade, or sharp object used.

Confirm

- Confirm the method of patient transfer due to positioning to minimize patient injury related to the type of procedure.
- Confirm that all equipment specific to the procedure is available and in the perioperative suite.

Evaluate and Ensure

- Evaluate the need for blood transfusion products, radiology personnel, blood salvage technical support, special instrumentation and equipment, and specialty OR table.
- Evaluate the need for warmed fluids, irrigants, and forced-air warming to promote normothermia.

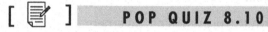

[📝]   POP QUIZ 8.10

An 80-year-old female presents to the OR for a cervical fusion following a motor vehicle crash involving three cars. The patient is hypertensive and has a history of myocardial infarction that occurred 7 years prior. The patient is anesthetized, positioned, prepped, and draped. What type of trauma is this, and what should the circulating nurse do next?

- Ensure all necessary equipment is available and that personnel associated with the procedure are in the surgical suite and ready to receive the patient.
- Ensure that the following are operational: equipment for the procedure, OR table and positioning equipment, oxygen supply and tanks, and suction.
- Ensure that the trauma team time-out is performed and includes the following: arrival situation report on the patient(s) and briefing to the team by the leader; prioritization of the patient needs based upon the assessment; report of the number of inbound patients; summary of the treatment; and team debrief.

RESOURCES

American Association of Nurse Anesthesiology. (2018). *Latex allergy management.* https://www.aana.com/docs/default-source/practice-aana-com-web-documents-(all)/professional-practice-manual/latex-allergy -management.pdf?sfvrsn=9c0049b1_8

American Society of Regional Anesthesia and Pain Medicine. (2020). *Checklist for treatment of local anesthetic systemic toxicity.* https://www.asra.com/guidelines-articles/guidelines/guideline-item/guidelines/2020/11/01/ checklist-for-treatment-of-local-anesthetic-systemic-toxicity

Apfelbaum, J. L., Hagberg, C. A., Caplan, R. A., Blitt, C. D., Connis, R. T., Nickinovich, D. G., & Hagberg, C. A. (2013). Practice guidelines for management of the difficult airway: An updated report by the American Society of Anesthesiologists Task Force on management of the difficult airway. *Anesthesiology, 118*(2), 251–270. https:// doi.org/10.1097/ALN.0b013e31827773b2

Association of periOperative Registered Nurses. (2021a). *Environment of care. Recommendation 3, guidelines for perioperative practice*. Author.

Association of periOperative Registered Nurses. (2021b). *EP4 verifying medication labels (NPSG.01.01.01)*. https://www.aornguidelines.org/joint-commission/program/46082/standard/46089/ep/543411

Association of periOperative Registered Nurses. (2021c). *Environment of care. Recommendation 4, guidelines for perioperative practice*. Author.

Association of periOperative Registered Nurses. (2021d). *Environment of care. Recommendation 5, guidelines for perioperative practice*. Author.

Association of periOperative Registered Nurses. (2021e). *Environment of care. Recommendation 7, guidelines for perioperative practice*. Author.

Association of periOperative Registered Nurses. (2021f). *Environment of care. Recommendation 8, guidelines for perioperative practice*. Author.

Association of periOperative Registered Nurses. (2021g). *Environment of care. Recommendation 10, guidelines for perioperative practice*. Author.

Association of periOperative Registered Nurses. (2021h). *Environment of care. Recommendation 11, guidelines for perioperative practice*. Author.

Association of periOperative Registered Nurses. (2021i). *Laser safety: Recommendation 1—precautions to mitigate hazards, guidelines for perioperative practice*. Author.

Association of periOperative Registered Nurses. (2021j). *Local anesthesia. Recommendation 3, guidelines for perioperative practice*. Author.

Association of periOperative Registered Nurses. (2021k). *Patient skin antisepsis, guidelines for perioperative practice*. Author.

Association of Surgical Technologists. (2018). *Guidelines for best practices for treatment of anaphylactic reaction in the surgical patient*. https://www.ast.org/uploadedFiles/Main_Site/Content/About_Us/Guideline_Anaphylactic_Reaction.pdf

Berkeley, A. V., Ahmed, M. F., & Reardon, J. M. (2021, July 23). *Anaphylaxis in the operating room*. Medscape. https://emedicine.medscape.com/article/2500072-overview

Carlos, G., & Saulan, M. (2018). Robotic emergencies: Are you prepared for a disaster? *AORN Journal, 108*(5), 493–501. https://doi.org/10.1002/aorn.12393

Feldheim, T., Lobo, S., Mallett, J. W., & Le-Wendling, L. (2021). *Local anesthetic systemic toxicity (LAST): A problem-based learning discussion*. https://www.asra.com/guidelines-articles/original-articles/article-item/legacy-b-blog-posts/2021/02/01/local-anesthetic-systemic-toxicity-(last)-a-problem-based-learning-discussion

Fitzgerald, M., Reilly, S., Smit, D. V., Kim, Y., Mathew, J., Boo, E., Alqahtani, A., Chowdhury, S., Darez, A., Mascarenhas, J. B., O'Keeffe, F., Noonan, M., Nickson, C., Marquez, M., Li, W. A., Zhang, Y. L., Williams, K., & Mitra, B. (2019). The World Health Organization trauma checklist versus trauma team time-out: A perspective. *Emergency Medicine Australasia, 31*(5), 882–885. https://doi.org/10.1111/1742-6723.13306

Franklin, B. (1735, February 4). *Protection of towns from fire*. The Pennsylvania Gazette.

Garvey, L. H., Dewachter, P., Hepner, D. L., Mertes, P. M., Voltolini, S., Clarke, R., Cooke, P., Garcez, T., Guttormsen, A. B., Ebo, D. G., Hopkins, P. M., Khan, D. A., Kopac, P., Krøigaard, M., Laguna, J. J., Marshall, S., Platt, P., Rose, M., Sabato, V., . . . Kolawole, H. (2019). Management of suspected immediate perioperative allergic reactions: An international overview and consensus recommendations. *British Journal of Anaesthesia Management, 123*(1), E50–E64. https://doi.org/10.1016/j.bja.2019.04.044

Kollmeier, B. R., Boyette, L. C., Beecham, G. B., Desai, N. M., Khetarpal, S. (2021, August 15). Difficult airway. *StatPearls*. StatPearls Publishing. https://www.ncbi.nlm.nih.gov/books/NBK470224

Malignant Hyperthermia Association of the United States. (2021). *MHAUS recommendations*. https://www.mhaus.org/healthcare-professionals/mhaus-recommendations

Neal, J. M., Neal, E. J., & Weinberg, G. L. (2021). American Society of Regional Anesthesia and Pain Medicine local anesthetic systemic toxicity checklist: 2020 version. *Regional Anesthesia & Pain Medicine, 46*(1), 81–82. https://doi.org/10.1136/rapm-2020-101986

Occupational Safety and Health Administration. (n.d.). *Surgical suite: Common safety and health topics.* U.D. Department of Labor, Occupational Safety and Health Administration. https://www.osha.gov/SLTC/etools/hospital/surgical/surgical.html

Rothrock, J. C. (Ed.). (2019). *Alexander's care of the patient in surgery* (16th ed.). Elsevier Health Sciences Division.

9 PROFESSIONAL ACCOUNTABILITY

OVERVIEW

- Society deems nurses accountable both individually and collectively for delivering quality care.
- The nurse, as a professional, is expected to provide exemplary care beyond the "it's just a job" mentality.
- Nursing as a profession requires the nurse's continuous engagement in professional development to demonstrate a personal commitment to delivering quality care above the expected standard.

ETHICAL AND PROFESSIONAL STANDARDS

Perioperative nurses adhere to the ethical guidelines and professional standards put forth by the American Nurses Association (ANA) and the Association of periOperative Registered Nurses (AORN).

American Nurses Association Code of Ethics

According to the ANA *Code of Ethics for Nurses, account-ability* is the professional responsibility that an individual nurse has for the patient, public, and healthcare organization to follow the scope and standards of nursing practice.

[✦]　　　　　　　　　**ALERT!**

The premise of safety culture is that systems, not individuals, are to blame for healthcare errors. Promoting a culture of safety balances delivering quality care at the required standard with holding individuals accountable when there is a conscious deviation from the standard.

Association of periOperative Registered Nurses Standards of Perioperative Nursing and the American Nurses Association Code of Ethics Alignment

- AORN's perioperative explications align with the ANA Code of Ethics.
- The Code of Ethics Interpretive Statements are as follows: 1.1 Respect for Human Dignity, 1.2 Relationship to Patients, 1.3 Nature of Health Problems, 1.4 Right to Self-Determination, 1.5 Relationships With Colleagues and Others, 2.1 Primacy of Patient Interest, 2.2 Conflict of Interest for Nurses, 2.3 Collaboration, 2.4 Professional Boundaries, 3.1 Privacy, 3.2 Confidentiality, 3.3 Protection of Participants in Research, 3.4 Standards and Review Mechanisms, 3.5 Acting on Questionable Practice, 3.6 Addressing Impaired Practice, 4.1 Acceptance of Accountability and Responsibility, 4.2 Accountability for Nursing Judgment and Action, 4.3 Responsibility for Nursing Judgment and Action, 4.4 Delegation of Nursing Activities, 5.1 Moral Self-Respect, 5.2 Professional Growth and Maintenance of Competency, 5.3 Wholeness of Character, 5.4 Preservation of Integrity, 6.1 Influence of the Environment on Moral Virtues and Values, 6.2 Influence of the Environment on Ethical Obligations, 6.3 Responsibility for Healthcare Environment, 7.1 Advancing the Profession, 8.1 Health as a Universal Right, 8.2 Collaboration for Health and Human Rights, and 9.1 Assertion of Values.

[📝]　　　　　　　　**POP QUIZ 9.1**

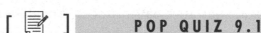

A 75-year-old patient is transported to the surgical suite for a right hip arthroplasty. During the administration of spinal anesthesia, the nurse takes steps to keep the patient covered. Which of the ANA Code of Ethics actions is the perioperative nurse observing?

NURSING SCOPE OF PRACTICE REQUIREMENTS

- Perioperative nursing scope of practice requirements align with practice requirements issued by the ANA Standards for Excellence, Scope and Standards of Practice, and the AORN-recommended practices.
- Perioperative nursing scope of practice requirements are patient centered and ascribe to a model of care that has four domains.

American Nurses Association Standards for Excellence

- The ANA's core message is that nurses should practice to the fullest extent of their licensure and education to improve healthcare access and provide high-quality care to patients.
- The ANA Standards for Excellence is a national initiative used to promote the highest standards and includes the following categories: finance and operations; leadership; legal compliance and ethics; mission, strategy, and evaluation; public awareness, engagement, and advocacy; and resource development.

American Nurses Association Scope and Standard for Practice

- The ANA Scope and Standard for Practice is a list of standards associated with the competency level of nursing care through the use of critical thinking and the nursing process.
- The standards of professional performance are associated with nursing practice that is based in evidence, collaborative, culturally sensitive, effectively communicated, environmentally safe, ethical, high quality, and resource efficient.

Association of periOperative Registered Nurses Guidelines for Perioperative Practice

- AORN's guidelines are considered the gold standard in evidence-based recommended practices guiding the perioperative nurse in decision-making, providing patient care, and promoting workplace safety.
- The guidelines are updated annually and offer recommendations for practice, development of policies and procedures, and criteria for measuring the competency level of the perioperative nurse.

 ALERT!

The perioperative nurse should not delegate beyond the requirements outlined in the state nurse practice act.

Four Domains

- The perioperative patient-focused model has four domains: health system where the care is provided, patient safety, patient's behavior in response to the procedure, and patient's physiologic response to operative interventions and invasive procedures.

State Licensure and Nurse Practice Acts

- Individual states govern health professional licensure.
- Nurse practice acts are state laws governing nursing practice and providing patient care rules and regulations.
- Nurse practice acts by state can be found on the National Council of State Boards of Nursing (NCSBN) website.
- State legislatures pass nurse practice acts, which define the scope of practice. To protect the public, regulatory bodies then issue rules and regulations based on these laws.
- The board of nursing for each state enforces the rules and regulations of nurse practice acts.
- The perioperative nurse must maintain all licensing requirements for the state and adhere to the nurse practice acts associated with each state.

LEGAL AND ETHICAL GUIDELINES FOR PATIENT CARE

- The healthcare industry is highly regulated; therefore, healthcare organizations and individuals must understand and comply with individual state laws and regulations, many of which govern practices related to ethical dilemmas perioperative personnel may face.
- The perioperative nurse works to promote health equity and ensures ethical treatment for all patients.

Health Equity

Care of the patient in the perioperative setting should include the following:

- Consideration of the patient's values, beliefs, and lifestyle choice
- Justice and equal treatment regardless of socioeconomic status, race, education, culture, religion, or age
- Protection of patient's free will and right to choose
- Treatment without prejudice or bias

Perioperative Ethical Dilemmas and Legal Issues

- Perioperative ethical dilemmas are commonly associated with the following: conflict of interest between the nurse's beliefs and the surgery to be performed; conflicting expectations associated with the patient's needs and surgeon's preferences; pressure to turn over a room faster; and witnessing of the signature on informed consent.
- There are four major categories of legal issues that may arise concerning perioperative nursing practice: organ donation and transplantation, quality of life, reproductive, and research.

Factors Contributing to Legal Issues

Factors contributing to legal issues in the perioperative setting include, but are not limited to, the following:

- Causing a direct patient injury related to deviation from duty or standard of care
- Delivery of a low standard of care
- Deviation from a standard of care or omission of important nursing interventions

Legal and Ethical Benefits Associated With Effective Documentation

- The perioperative nurse has a duty to accurately document all aspects of patient care during the three phases of the perioperative process, ensure that all patient medical information is protected, and safeguard the electronic health record or other charting modality by exiting the record and safely filing its contents.
- The permanent legal record should be created using a standardized format and incorporate the use of the standardized terminology provided by the perioperative nursing data set (PNDS).

PROMOTING A CULTURE OF SAFETY

- All members of the perioperative team must work to promote a culture of safety.
- National guidelines and recommendations help organizations achieve this goal.
- The ANA Code of Ethics, AORN Guidelines, The Joint Commission (TJC) standards, and engagement on committees and professional organizations contribute to the professional development of the nurse and assist in promoting a culture of safety.

The Nurse's Role in Promoting a Culture of Safety

- AORN's (2015c) *Position Statement on a Healthy Perioperative Practice Environment* requires an organization to promote the following: accountability among all team members; collaborative practice; communication that is respectful, helpful, and useful; encouragement of professional practice; recognition of the contributions made by nursing; shared decision-making; and the visibility of expert leadership.
- The perioperative nurse can promote a culture of safety by doing the following: accurately interpreting the patient's identity and the procedure to be performed; ensuring all surgical counts are performed according to facility policy to reduce the risk of retained foreign bodies; handling all surgical instrumentation and equipment in a safe manner to prevent injury to the patient or the surgical team members; handling patient's personal property with care and ensuring that all personal effects are safely secured per facility policy; promoting a culture of respect, collaboration, and teamwork; protecting the patient from accidental fall or injury during transport to the surgical suite and transfer to the surgical table by ensuring adequate personnel are available to assist; reporting all adverse events and changes to the patient's condition; and safely securing and preparing all specimens per facility policy.

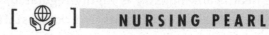

[🌐]   NURSING PEARL

Use the mnemonic **CCARES** to remember how to promote a culture of safety:

- Collaborate with the team.
- Communicate effectively.
- Accept responsibility for your actions.
- Recognize the contributions of others.
- Encourage one another.
- Share in the decision-making.

American Nurses Association Code of Ethics

- The ANA *Code of Ethics for Nurses With Interpretative Statements* calls upon employers in both academic and clinical settings to foster a workplace free of incivility, lateral and workplace violence, and bullying.
- The perioperative nurse has a responsibility to the self and others to use best practices related to the management and report of issues associated with incivility, lateral or workplace violence, and bullying, including the following: collaborate with all team members through open dialogue and sharing of information in a timely manner; encourage a nonpunitive work environment; maintain a detailed written account of incidents; participate in workplace violence prevention education programs and postevent debriefings; provide assistance when needed; recognize one's own actions in a situation; rely on facts and refrain from spreading gossip or rumors; remain open to the ideas of others; respond to incivility in a respectful manner and report using the appropriate channels; support team members who have been a target of uncivil behaviors or workplace violence; treat all team members with respect and dignity; use clear and civil communication across all mediums (written, verbal, social media, etc.); and work to incorporate personal wellness strategies to decrease stress.

Association of periOperative Registered Nurses Recommendations

- AORN recommends that organizational leadership should implement best practices to promote a safety culture. Best practices should promote respect, honesty, collaboration, and accountability among individuals and teams across healthcare disciplines. They should also facilitate effective communication and empower perioperative personnel to speak up. Examples include the following: interdisciplinary team members participate in a standardized approach to hand-off communication, including verification using readback methods; perioperative personnel comply with the protocol for patient preprocedure checks and time-out processes, and each team member participates and contributes. ▶

Association of periOperative Registered Nurses Recommendations (*continued*)

■ AORN encourages employers to offer structured orientation as a means to encourage a safety culture. Perioperative residency programs assist in decreasing the theory-to-practice gap and should include preceptor education, training, and evaluation. Precepted competency-based orientation programs should be measurable and provided to perioperative RNs and surgical technologists upon hire.

The Joint Commission Standards

■ TJC highlights key standards integral to an organization's commitment to safety culture.

■ TJC issues National Patient Safety Goals (NPSGs) annually to highlight healthcare-related adverse events and practice issues in the following practice areas: ambulatory healthcare, behavioral healthcare, critical access hospital, home care, hospital, laboratory, nursing care center, and office-based surgery center.

■ The following are NPSGs associated with the perioperative setting: identifying patient safety risks, identifying patients correctly, improving staff communication, preventing infection, preventing mistakes in surgery, safety associated with medication administration, and utilization of alarms.

■ These standards from TJC require that the organizational leadership implement the following practices: nonpunitive internal mechanisms for reporting near or actual adverse events to encourage reporting and increase opportunities for shared learning; policies that prohibit intimidating behaviors; procedures for promoting a safety culture and performing assessments through the use of validated surveys to identify areas for improvement; and risk assessment approaches emphasizing that systems, not individuals, are to blame for near or actual events.

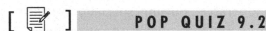

POP QUIZ 9.2

A circulating nurse contributes to a medication error. The circulating nurse reports the mistake through the safety event system. An root cause anaylsis (RCA) ensues. The collaborative RCA findings point to an inadequate electronic medical record fail-safe mechanism for alerting healthcare professionals to overdose or underdose medication. The processes described in this scenario illustrate which key concepts around safety culture?

PROFESSIONAL GROWTH AND ACCOUNTABILITY

■ Ongoing engagement in professional growth and accountability is a foundational aspect of nursing practice.

■ Maintaining personal accountability to the self and others, participating in membership in national organizations, obtaining specialty certification, and engaging in professional development activities are ways that the perioperative nurse can grow professionally.

Accountability

AORN highlights the professional practice of the perioperative RN within the context of accountability to illustrate the importance of a nurse's behavior. The RN is accountable to the patient, team, and organization for performing at a level that is considered the standard of care.

■ Perioperative leadership teams have moral and legal responsibilities to identify risks and implement actions to prevent harm.

■ Perioperative nursing is a specialty that requires ongoing professional development to continually increase knowledge and skills.

■ Perioperative personnel who lack accountability for behavior may cause patient harm and patient dissatisfaction with the quality of care.

Membership in National Organizations

AORN encourages membership in professional organizations. These associations provide evidence-based guidelines and standards for patient safety and clinical issues. Examples of professional organizations in which nurses may seek membership include the following:

- ANA: https://www.nursingworld.org/membership/joinANA
- American Society of PeriAnesthesia Nurses (ASPAN): https://www.aspan.org
- Association for Nursing Professional Development (ANPD): https://www.anpd.org
- Association of Professionals in Infection Control and Epidemiology (APIC): https://apic.org
- AORN: https://www.aorn.org
- National League of Nursing (NLN): http://www.nln.org
- Healthcare Sterile Processing Association (HSPA): https://myhspa.org

Professional Development

- AORN strongly encourages professional development and specifically endorses the value of specialty certification.
- Perioperative nursing specialty certification demonstrates to the public, patients, colleagues, and employers that nurses are committed to delivering the highest quality care possible. Perioperative nursing specialty certification is a formal means to recognize nurses' knowledge, skills, and experience; it measures the nurse's knowledge objectively, validating at a standard level the knowledge necessary to provide high-quality care. Perioperative leadership teams should display the credentials of certified perioperative RNs; market the RNs' professional certification to the public to demonstrate alignment with AORN's message of seeking licensure, accreditation, certification, and education to promote patient safety and provide protection to the public; and support RNs in obtaining certification.
- The perioperative nurse should utilize the resources available at the place of work, in the community, and through professional organizations to enhance professional growth.

QUALITY IMPROVEMENT USING EVIDENCE-BASED PRACTICE

The perioperative nurse should remain engaged in quality improvement initiatives and incorporate the use of evidence-based practice guidelines and recommendations in all facets of practice.

Engagement in Evidence-Based Practice

Evidence-based practices are the foundation of the AORN guidelines. Perioperative personnel should use the guidelines to inform quality patient care and quality improvement strategies, including the implementation of policies based on best practices. Examples include standardization in the following areas:

- Counting process
- Hand-off approach
- Patient identification
- Patient normothermia protocols
- Time-out processes

Quality Improvement Agencies

Quality improvement agencies decrease healthcare costs, enhance provider experience, and improve population health, patient experiences, or patient outcomes. Quality improvement agencies include the following: ▶

Quality Improvement Agencies (*continued*)

- Agency for Healthcare Research and Quality
- Institute for Healthcare Improvement
- TJC Center for Transforming Healthcare

Methods for Quality Improvement Engagement

- Common process or quality improvement models used in the perioperative setting include, but are not limited to, the following: **PICO** framework for developing clinical questions: Plan-Do-Study-Act; RCA; and Six Sigma.
- Participation in quality-of-care activities helps the perioperative nurse to stay engaged and promote lasting change by advocating for changes to processes that impede a safe and effective workflow; attending meetings and serving on committees related to quality improvement initiatives; collecting data on quality improvement initiatives; identifying and accepting responsibility for ongoing monitoring and evaluation activities within the department; maintaining knowledge on current practice changes, professional nursing scope of practice responsibilities, delegation restraints, and regulatory standards; and performing quality assessments and RCAs on a routine basis.
- Shared governance fosters quality improvement engagement for the perioperative nurse by empowering nurses to continuously improve patient care and the work environment; enhancing collaboration with interprofessional team members to improve patient care; and providing nurses with responsibility, authority, and accountability related to decision-making processes.

RESOURCES

Agency for Healthcare Research and Quality. (n.d.). *Patient safety and quality improvement.* https://www.ahrq.gov/patient-safety/index.html

American Nurses Association. (2015a). *American Nurses Association position statement on incivility, bullying, and workplace violence.* https://www.nursingworld.org/~49d6e3/globalassets/practiceandpolicy/nursing-excellence/incivility-bullying-and-workplace-violence--ana-position-statement.pdf

American Nurses Association. (2015b). *Code of ethics for nurses with interpretive statements.* https://www.nursingworld.org/practice-policy/nursing-excellence/ethics/code-of-ethics-for-nurses/coe-view-only

American Nurses Association. (n.d.). *Scope of practice.* https://www.nursingworld.org/practice-policy/scope-of-practice

Association of periOperative Registered Nurses. (2015a). *Exhibit A: Historical perspectives on the AORN standards, competency statements, and certification. AORN standards.* https://www.aorn.org/guidelines/clinical-resources/aorn-standards

Association of periOperative Registered Nurses. (2015b). *Healthy perioperative practice environment. Position statements.* https://www.aorn.org/guidelines/clinical-resources/position-statements

Association of periOperative Registered Nurses. (2015c). *Position statement on a healthy perioperative practice environment. Position statements.* https://www.aorn.org/guidelines/clinical-resources/position-statements

Association of periOperative Registered Nurses. (2016). *Perioperative nursing certification. Position statements.* https://www.aorn.org/guidelines/clinical-resources/position-statements

Association of periOperative Registered Nurses. (2017). *AORN's perioperative explications for the ANA code of ethics for nurses with interpretative statements.* https://www.aorn.org/guidelines/clinical-resources/code-of-ethics

Association of periOperative Registered Nurses. (2018). *Position statement on orientation of the registered nurse and surgical technologist to the perioperative setting. Position statements.* https://www.aorn.org/guidelines/clinical-resources/position-statements

Association of periOperative Registered Nurses. (2019). *AORN position statement on perioperative registered nurse residency programs. Position statements.* https://www.aorn.org/guidelines/clinical-resources/position-statements

Association of periOperative Registered Nurses. (2021a). *About: Guidelines for perioperative practice.* https://www.aorn.org/guidelines/about-aorn-guidelines

Association of periOperative Registered Nurses. (2021b). *Guideline for a safe environment of care, guidelines for perioperative practice.* Author.

Clement, N. (2013). *Ethical and legal issues in perioperative nursing. Nursing ethics.* Pearson India. https://learning.oreilly.com/library/view/nursing-ethics/9788131773345/xhtml/chapter030.xhtml

Institute for Healthcare Improvement. (n.d.). *Quality improvement essentials toolkit.* [Toolkit]. http://www.ihi.org/resources/Pages/Tools/Quality-Improvement-Essentials-Toolkit.aspx

The Joint Commission. (2018). *Patient safety systems. Comprehensive accreditation manual.* Joint Commission Resources.

The Joint Commission Center for Transforming Healthcare. (n.d.). *Who we are.* https://www.centerfortransforminghealthcare.org/who-we-are/

Kutney-Lee, A., Germack, H., Hatfield, L., Kelly, S., Maguire, P., Dierkes, A., Guidice, M. D., & Aiken, L. H. (2016). Nurse engagement in shared governance and patient and nurse outcomes. *The Journal of Nursing Administration, 46*(11), 605–612. https://doi.org/10.1097/NNA.0000000000000412

Rothrock, J. C. (Ed.). (2019). *Alexander's care of the patient in surgery* (16th ed.). Elsevier Health Sciences Division.

10 PRACTICE TEST QUESTIONS

1. Which of the following terminates the direct perioperative nurse–patient relationship?
   A. Completion of surgery
   B. The follow-up phone call
   C. When the patient leaves the post-anesthesia care unit (PACU)
   D. When the patient enters Phase II of the PACU

2. The nurse is cleaning up at the bedside of the patient after administering an intramuscular injection for pain, then changes the bandage on an abdominal postoperative incision. The nurse will dispose of the syringe with needle, saturated bloody gauze, and bloody scissors into what type of waste receptacle?
   A. Biohazard bag
   B. Non-biohazard bag
   C. Sharps container
   D. Non-biohazard container

3. Which intraoperative communication is an environmental barrier?
   A. Social talk
   B. Standardized
   C. Closed-loop
   D. Structured

4. The overall goal of preoperative assessment is to:
   A. Collect the patient's data
   B. Determine the patient's goal for surgery
   C. Address risk factors that might delay recovery
   D. Ensure all necessary diagnostic tests are performed and checklists completed

5. Which of the following is a late sign of malignant hyperthermia?
   A. Myoglobinuria
   B. Tachycardia
   C. Muscle rigidity
   D. Tachypnea

6. On-call staffing schedules support a healthy work environment by:
   A. Maximizing overtime use and allowing recuperation time between work hours
   B. Maximizing overtime use and allowing team members to set their own schedule
   C. Minimizing overtime use and allowing recuperation time between work hours
   D. Minimizing overtime use and allowing team members to set their own schedule

7. What is the time frame in which frozen sections should be processed for pathology?
   A. 0 to 5 minutes
   B. 10 to 20 minutes
   C. 30 to 60 minutes
   D. 45 to 60 minutes

8. The nurse places a patient in supine position with legs uncrossed to prevent:
   A. Skin breakdown
   B. Surgical drapes from being uneven
   C. Injury to the lower back
   D. Cutting off circulation in the lower extremities

9. Which of the following components of the preoperative checklist for surgery are considered essential?
   A. Patient identification, operative consent, allergies
   B. Patient address, chest x-ray results, urine output
   C. Patient insurance information, personal effects, lab results
   D. Patient assigned room after surgery, family contact information

10. To assess potential illicit drug use in a preoperative patient, the perioperative nurse would:
    A. Ask a family member of the patient
    B. Ask the patient in a frank, direct manner
    C. Ask the patient to fill out a questionnaire
    D. Assume the patient does not use illicit drugs and omit that line of questioning

11. Which of the following provides standards for the reduction of exposure to noxious stimuli?
    A. National Quality Forum
    B. Centers for Disease Control and Prevention
    C. American National Standards Institute
    D. National Fire Protection Association

12. The circulating nurse and scrub person are setting up the OR for an afternoon surgery. The nurse is positioning the bed under the overhead light fixture. The scrub person asks the nurse to move the anesthesia equipment into the proper place and check the connections. The circulating nurse's BEST response is:
    A. "The anesthesia equipment is moved last to ensure the other supplies have ample room."
    B. "That is not my responsibility; you should move it."
    C. "We are not trained to move the anesthesia equipment. Only the anesthesiologist can do that."
    D. "The anesthesia equipment does not need to be moved. The room is set up to accommodate it."

13. Supply costs typically make up what percentage of the total operating room budget?
    A. 15%
    B. 25%
    C. 56%
    D. 86%

14. The nurse has concluded a preoperative medical history and physical assessment and is analyzing the data to formulate a nursing diagnosis. The priority problem for the patient is a history of a mild-to-moderate reaction to bananas and kiwi. This places the patient at an increased risk for allergy to:
    A. Antimicrobial infusions
    B. Latex products
    C. Corticosteroid injections
    D. Metal instruments

15. A patient preparing for surgery wishes not to be intubated. The nurse documents their code status as:
    A. Do not resuscitate (DNR)
    B. Do not intubate (DNI)
    C. Full Code
    D. DNR/DNI

16. The appropriate airflow for decontamination and sterilizer equipment is:
    A. Positive
    B. Negative
    C. Neutral
    D. It does not matter

17. Which role is the experienced nurse practicing when recognizing the need to cultivate an environment of growth in clinical practice for novice nurses?
    A. Mentor
    B. Advocate
    C. Preceptor
    D. Manager

18. The primary purpose of terminal cleaning is to:
    A. Control air particle exposure
    B. Control the spread of infection
    C. Control the use of disinfectants
    D. Control the use of sterilization

19. A patient who received an injection of a ropivacaine mixture for shoulder surgery begins to convulse and stop breathing. The nurse's BEST next action is to:
    A. Administer propofol
    B. Administer lorazepam
    C. Administer lipid emulsion
    D. Administer norepinephrine bitartrate

20. According to the Association of periOperative Registered Nurses position statement on environmental responsibility, perioperative surgical settings account for what percentage of the facility's total waste?
    A. Close to three quarters
    B. Nearly all
    C. Close to half
    D. Less than a quarter

21. An appendectomy performed for acute, unruptured appendicitis is classified as which type of wound?
    A. Class I
    B. Class II
    C. Class III
    D. Class IV

22. The postoperative nurse assesses a patient with lip swelling, shortness of breath, and rhinitis. The nurse's BEST initial action is to:
    A. Notify the anesthesiologist
    B. Administer 0.9% sodium chloride infusion
    C. Administer 100% oxygen
    D. Administer a corticosteroid

23. The primary reason the nurse should assess a patient's kidney function before surgery is to determine:
    A. Excretion ability
    B. Tolerance for a urinary catheter
    C. Presence of a urinary infection
    D. Patient's ability to urinate independently

24. What is the MOST common cause of delayed wound healing in surgical patients?
    A. Immunocompromised status
    B. Diabetes
    C. Smoking
    D. Surgical site infection

25. The Association of periOperative Registered Nurses position statement on environmental responsibility recommends reducing waste by utilizing reprocessing of what type of device?
    A. Double-use device
    B. Triple-use device
    C. Implant device
    D. Single-use device

26. A fire breaks out in the OR. The surgical team's INITIAL action is to:
    A. Find the source of the fire
    B. Stop the flow of all airway gases
    C. Smother the fire with blankets
    D. Remove the patient from the OR

27. The nurse is conducting a preoperative assessment on a patient who will be undergoing above-the-knee amputation. The patient plainly states, "I will no longer be able to walk by myself." Which of the following is the MOST appropriate nursing diagnosis?
    A. Powerlessness
    B. Ineffective coping
    C. Anticipatory grieving
    D. Risk for disturbed body image

28. Which diagnostic marker is considered highly sensitive in diagnosing anaphylaxis?
    A. Histamine
    B. Tryptase level
    C. Intradermal test
    D. Skin prick test

29. The circulating nurse is participating in an aortic valve replacement. An artery was nicked and blood got all over the instrument towel. The nurse's BEST action is to:
    A. Remove the blood-soaked towel and replace it with a new sterile towel
    B. Leave the towel alone; it does not need to be changed out
    C. Leave the towel where it is and place a new sterile towel over it
    D. Obtain a new Mayo stand and replace all the instruments and towels

30. The nurse who is working to improve healthcare at local, state, and national levels of government is advocating for changes in:
    A. Standards
    B. Guidelines
    C. Policy
    D. Protocols

31. The nurse is performing a preoperative assessment and reviews the patient's lab levels: Potassium level 2.0 mEq/L, sodium 130 mEq/L, fasting blood glucose 95 mg/dL. The nurse's BEST action is to:
    A. Contact the surgeon to hold the surgery
    B. Start 0.9% of NaCl and prepare for surgery
    C. Administer 1 amp of D50 and prepare for surgery
    D. Document the labs on the surgical checklist and send to surgery

32. Which of the following may contribute to a novice nurse lacking knowledge in the surgical setting?
    A. No exposure to perioperative patient care in nursing curriculum
    B. Minimal exposure to perioperative patient care in nursing curriculum
    C. Minimal interest in perioperative patient care by nursing instructors
    D. No interest in mentorships by management for perioperative patient care

33. The nurse is caring for a trauma patient and suspects that the patient is developing venous thromboembolism. Which of the following findings leads the nurse to suspect this diagnosis?
   A. Charcot's triad
   B. Virchow's triad
   C. Beck's triad
   D. Cushing's triad

34. What personal protective equipment should the nurse wear in the decontamination area?
   A. Mask, goggles, long-cuffed utility gloves, double gown, shoe covers
   B. Mask, face shield, two pairs of regular gloves, gown, shoe covers
   C. Head covering, face shield, long-cuffed utility gloves, gown, shoe covers
   D. Head covering, mask, goggles, two pairs of regular gloves, gown, shoe covers

35. The surgeon requests a thin radiopaque latex drain. The nurse hands the surgeon a:
   A. Foley catheter
   B. Penrose drain
   C. Hemovac
   D. Jackson Pratt

36. What should a nurse do when receiving a phone order?
   A. Repeat it back before hanging up
   B. Tell the provider they cannot take a telephone order
   C. Write the order on a sheet of paper for the provider to input later
   D. Ask the pharmacist to clarify the accuracy of the order

37. A natural disaster has occurred in the surrounding community and a disaster code has been issued. The nurse manager calls the disaster team members to report to the facility to implement the plan of care. This process is known as:
   A. Disaster recall
   B. Filtration zone
   C. Reverse triage
   D. Surge capacity

38. The nurse is communicating with a patient during the perioperative phase. Which of the following elements is MOST critical for the nurse to remember?
   A. To repeat all information stated
   B. To hold all communications in strict confidentiality
   C. To appropriately document all answers given by the patient
   D. To ask difficult questions in a direct and frank manner

39. Which of the following commonly used surgical procedures is most likely to cause the release of gaseous byproducts from surgical smoke?
    A. Electrocautery ablation and radiation ablation
    B. Electrocautery ablation and laser ablation
    C. Radiation ablation and laser ablation
    D. Radiation ablation and cryoablation

40. During the preoperative assessment, a patient exhibits high levels of anxiety. The nurse educates the patient on how to use imagery, distraction, and self-recitation to reduce their anxiety. These are examples of _____ coping strategies.
    A. Affective
    B. Psychomotor
    C. Cognitive
    D. Physical

41. The intraoperative nurse is monitoring a patient's heart rhythm on the monitor. It shows three ventricular beats in a row, at a rate of 120 bpm. The nurse recognizes that the patient is in:
    A. Sinus tachycardia
    B. Ventricular fibrillation
    C. Ventricular tachycardia
    D. Pulseless electrical activity

42. The nurse has completed the preoperative assessment when the patient notes that they do not wish to be resuscitated. The nurse will request an order for:
    A. Patient clearance for surgery
    B. A do not resuscitate
    C. Surgery postponement
    D. Surgery cancellation

43. What two organizations have issued hand hygiene guidelines that should be followed to promote the reduction of healthcare-associated infections?
    A. World Health Organization and Centers for Disease Control and Prevention
    B. World Health Organization and Centers for Medicare and Medicaid Services
    C. Centers for Medicare and Medicaid Services and Centers for Disease Control and Prevention
    D. Centers for Medicare and Medicaid Services and The Joint Commission

44. A new perioperative nurse asks a more experienced nurse to explain the debriefing process. The nurse's MOST appropriate response is:
    A. "How long have you been in perioperative care?"
    B. "How long have you been out of nursing school?"
    C. "What do you know about debriefing?"
    D. "I will tell you where to access information on the debriefing process."

45. An example of mechanical hemostasis is:
   A. Tourniquet
   B. Fibrin glue
   C. Electrosurgery unit
   D. Laser

46. A patient during surgery has a rapid increase in their core temperature, and arterial blood gases indicate mixed respiratory and metabolic acidosis. The anesthetic agent is discontinued and the patient is placed on 100% oxygen. The nurse will prepare to administer:
   A. Tizanidine
   B. Dantrolene
   C. Metaxalone
   D. Methocarbamol

47. The nurse has just started a propofol infusion on a patient who was administered a local anesthetic mixture. The patient starts to convulse, becomes hypotensive, and remains in sinus rhythm. The nurse's NEXT action is to:
   A. Remove the propofol
   B. Administer lorazepam
   C. Start a lipid emulsion infusion
   D. Administer norepinephrine bitartrate

48. A nurse in preoperative care is preparing a 9-year-old boy for surgery. His mother is at the bedside and tells the nurse the child is very worried about having a catheter inserted. What is the appropriate response by the nurse?
   A. "Don't worry. It doesn't hurt."
   B. "You signed the consent form, so he has to have it."
   C. "He has to have a catheter, so he's going to have to be brave."
   D. "The catheter is inserted during surgery, so you won't feel it."

49. Which of the following conditions is caused by the development of microthrombi in smaller blood vessels?
   A. Rhabdomyolysis
   B. Hemorrhage
   C. Hypoxemia
   D. Disseminated intravascular coagulation

50. The sterility assurance level is the:
   A. Amount of time it takes for a sterilization process to kill 1 million microorganisms
   B. Mathematical expression of the time, temperature, and pressure required to kill microorganisms
   C. Number of microorganisms that are killed during the sterilization process
   D. Mathematical expression of the probability that an organism is present on an item after sterilization

51. Which organization provides standards and guidelines for perianesthesia?
    A. American Society of PeriAnesthesia Nurses
    B. Association for Professionals in Infection Control and Epidemiology
    C. Association for the Advancement of Medical Instrumentation
    D. International Association of Healthcare Central Service Materiel Management

52. Which of the following is an individual characteristic that may present barriers to effective team communication?
    A. Accent
    B. Time pressure
    C. Emotional stress
    D. Multitasking

53. The heat from a diathermy causes the rupture of cell membranes, which causes a plume of smoke to develop, resulting in what reaction?
    A. Release of gaseous byproducts into the body tissue
    B. Release of gaseous byproducts into the surgical instrument
    C. Release of gaseous byproducts into the atmosphere
    D. Release of gaseous byproducts into the patient

54. The basic rule of conduct between patients and members of a healthcare team within a medical facility is the:
    A. Code of Ethics
    B. Patient Bill of Rights
    C. Informed consent
    D. Consumer rights and protections

55. The Centers for Medicare and Medicaid Services guidelines state that verbal orders should:
    A. Never be given
    B. Be limited to emergency situations
    C. Be signed within 72 hours of being given
    D. Be documented by the nurse within 24 hours

56. Which of the following is a standardized communication tool used throughout the perioperative setting to promote patient safety among the surgical team?
    A. Electronic digital charting
    B. SBAR form
    C. Surgical safety checklist
    D. Incident report

57. What degree is required to become an RN first assistant?
    A. Associate degree in nursing
    B. Diploma degree in nursing
    C. Master's degree in nursing
    D. Bachelor's degree in nursing

58. The surgeon announces they are splitting. The nurse understands that:
    A. Blood and fluid will be removed from the surgical site
    B. Muscle will be separated along fascial layers
    C. Structures will be displaced using an instrument
    D. The flow of blood will be stopped

59. AMRA stands for:
    A. Adverse malignant reactions to anesthesia
    B. Adverse metabolic reactions to anesthesia
    C. Adverse monitoring of reactions to anesthesia
    D. Adverse management of reactions to anesthesia

60. Which antibiotic is the MOST common cause of anaphylaxis?
    A. Penicillin
    B. Ciprofloxacin
    C. Clindamycin
    D. Metronidazole

61. A surgical patient who just received a local anesthetic complains of ringing in their ears, lightheadedness, and blurred vision. The nurse suspects that the patient is experiencing:
    A. Syncope
    B. Meniere's disease
    C. Orthostatic hypotension
    D. Local anesthetic system toxicity

62. Using sharp or blunt methods to separate tissues is called:
    A. Dissection
    B. Harvesting
    C. Traction
    D. Procurement

63. Rapid sequence induction is an algorithm used by surgeons and anesthesiologists to prevent:
    A. Aspiration
    B. Pulmonary edema
    C. Laryngospasm
    D. Hemorrhage

64. Which diagnostic test is considered the gold standard for diagnosing malignant hyperthermia in the United States?
    A. Genetic testing
    B. DNA sampling
    C. In vitro contracture test
    D. Caffeine-halothane contracture test

65. The nurse discovers that a sponge is missing during a closing count for a left lung lobectomy. Which is the most appropriate INITIAL action by the nurse?
    A. Repeat the count
    B. Notify the surgeon
    C. Document the count as incorrect
    D. Notify the supervisor

66. Which surgical team member supplies the fuel source that may contribute to an operating fire?
    A. Surgeon
    B. Anesthesiologist
    C. Circulating nurse
    D. RN first assistant

67. The nurse is training a new hire who asks why they need to know how a patient reacted to anesthesia in the past. The nurse's BEST response is:
    A. Previous reactions will guide the medication selection for this surgery
    B. The previous reaction needs to be charted in the medical record
    C. The previous reaction could indicate an underlying allergy
    D. It's a matter of protocol

68. A patient is experiencing malignant hyperthermia. The surgical team's INITIAL action is to:
    A. Administer a muscle relaxant
    B. Administer sodium bicarbonate
    C. Discontinue triggering agents
    D. Hyperventilate with 100% oxygen

69. The circulating nurse is setting up the OR for a breast augmentation procedure and is placing supplies on the sterile field. The nurse flips the sutures onto the sterile field and the implants into a sterile basin. Which of the following is the MOST accurate statement regarding the nurse's actions?
    A. The nurse created a larger sterile field to accommodate the flipped sutures and implants
    B. While sutures can be flipped into the sterile field, implants should never be flipped
    C. While implants can be flipped into the sterile field, sutures should never be flipped
    D. Supplies should never be flipped into the sterile field, regardless of their size

70. What type of questioning method would the preoperative nurse use when performing a psychosocial assessment?
    A. Direct
    B. Probing
    C. Open-ended
    D. Closed-ended

71. What two areas should the perioperative team weigh when determining ideal patient positioning?
    A. Surgical comfort vs. risks related to patient position
    B. Surgical comfort vs. safety related to patient position
    C. Surgical comfort vs. knowledge of surgical procedure
    D. Surgical comfort vs. number of team members needed

72. What electrolyte imbalance increases the risk for cardiac arrest?
    A. Hyperkalemia
    B. Hypokalemia
    C. Hypermagnesemia
    D. Hypomagnesemia

73. The postoperative nurse is utilizing the situation, background, assessment, and recommendation (SBAR) method to call a report to the nurse who will be accepting the surgical patient. Which information will the nurse include in the "B" portion?
    A. Recommendations
    B. Vital signs
    C. Mental status
    D. Required tests

74. Which of the following completes the perioperative nursing process?
    A. When the patient recovers
    B. When the patient enters post-anesthesia care unit
    C. When the patient discharges
    D. When the patient enters the operating room

75. A circulating nurse yawns repeatedly during the briefing and the surgical time-out. What is the most appropriate action by the surgical team?
    A. Give the nurse a cup of coffee and continue the procedure
    B. Stop the procedure and reschedule for later in the day
    C. Ask the nurse to have another nurse relieve them of their duties
    D. Decrease the temperature in the room to keep the nurse alert

76. During an open abdominal hernia repair, the anesthesiologist announces that they need to decrease the patient's intracranial pressure. The circulating nurse will:
    A. Place the patient in Trendelenburg position
    B. Place the patient in reverse Trendelenburg position
    C. Place the patient in supine position
    D. Place the patient in prone position

77. The intraoperative nurse is preparing a patient with a body mass index (BMI) of 32 for a major surgical procedure. Based on this data, the nurse will ensure that which of the following is available in the OR?
    A. Ice packs and cooling blankets
    B. Mannitol
    C. Dantrolene
    D. Flexible laryngoscope

78. Which of the following provides guidance for the delegation of certain tasks to unlicensed assistive personnel?
    A. Medicare guidelines
    B. Patient Bill of Rights
    C. Scope of practice
    D. Licensure compact

79. A patient should discontinue aspirin use _____ prior to surgery.
    A. 24 hours
    B. 48 hours
    C. 3 to 4 days
    D. 7 to 10 days

80. The nurse is teaching a patient how to use an incentive spirometer postoperatively. Which of the following instructions does the nurse include?
    A. You should use it three times and repeat every 4 hours around the clock
    B. You should use it five times and repeat every 2 hours when you are awake
    C. You should use it five times and repeat every hour when you are awake
    D. You should use it 10 times and repeat every hour when you are awake

81. The perioperative nurse is explaining medical forms, informed consent, and HIPAA to a patient prior to surgery. The patient asks what HIPAA stands for. The nurse's response is:
    A. Health Insurance Portability and Availability Act
    B. Health Insurance Protection and Accountability Act
    C. Health Insurance Portability and Accountability Act
    D. Health Insurance Protection and Availability Act

82. Noise and distractions can potentially increase the adverse effects on patient care outcomes, initiate poor task performance, and promote a decreased ability to concentrate. This leads to what type of performance outcome for the surgical nurse?
    A. Inability to perform complex problem-solving tasks
    B. Inability to perform simple problem-solving tasks
    C. Ability to perform complex patient care tasks
    D. Ability to perform simple patient care tasks

83. The nurse is preparing a 75-year-old patient for transurethral resection of the prostate. The nurse is concerned about which of the following preoperative lab values?
    A. Hematocrit 48%
    B. Platelets 300,000/mcL
    C. Potassium 2.5 mEq/L
    D. White blood cells 8,000/mcL

84. What is the term that describes the period of time in which an item is considered sterile?
    A. Package life
    B. Condition life
    C. Shelf life
    D. Material life

85. What type of allergic reaction is anaphylaxis?
    A. Immune complex-type
    B. Cytotoxic-type
    C. Delayed-type
    D. Immediate-type

86. The American Nurses Association and Association of periOperative Registered Nurses have established joint guidelines for which element of patient care?
    A. Legal issues
    B. Ethical issues
    C. Financial issues
    D. Spiritual issues

87. Which of the following describes a wound that heals after primary union without further intervention?
    A. First-intention healing
    B. Second-intention healing
    C. Third-intention healing
    D. Delayed primary closure

88. What role is the nurse functioning in when the nursing process is utilized with the interdisciplinary team in all phases of the perioperative phases, but the nurse does not need to wear sterile attire?
    A. Scrub nurse
    B. Float nurse
    C. Circulating nurse
    D. Advanced practice nurse

89. The nurse is pouring liquids into a sterile surgical tray. Which of the following is considered sterile?
    A. Outer cap of pouring container
    B. Spraying fluid
    C. Inner cap of pouring container
    D. Entire pouring container

90. How many physical status classifications are included in the American Society of Anesthesiologists physical status classification scale?
    A. 3
    B. 6
    C. 10
    D. 8

91. To ensure that a patient understands their discharge instructions, the nurse will ask the patient to:
    A. Sign a form confirming that discharge instructions have been given
    B. Watch a video with discharge instructions
    C. Verbally confirm that they understand the instructions
    D. Repeat back important instructions

92. A patient immediately postoperative becomes unresponsive to the surgical team. A code is called, and CPR is initiated. The heart monitor reveals ventricular fibrillation. The nurse's INITIAL action is to:
    A. Resume CPR
    B. Check for a pulse
    C. Obtain IV access
    D. Deliver a shock

93. The situation, background, assessment, and recommendation (SBAR) tool is used to promote:
    A. Patient safety
    B. Confidentiality
    C. Infection control
    D. Pain control

94. During the preadmission assessment, a patient asks the nurse the same questions repeatedly. The patient also avoids eye contact. This patient is MOST LIKELY experiencing:
    A. Anxiety
    B. Depression
    C. Powerlessness
    D. A knowledge deficit

95. The perioperative nurse manager has been involved with maintaining standards of care while also preparing for the accreditation review by The Joint Commission. Which tool does the nurse manager use to ensure survey-readiness?
    A. The Association of periOperative Registered Nurses Accreditation Code
    B. The Association of periOperative Registered Nurses Accreditation Checklist
    C. The Association of periOperative Registered Nurses Accreditation Assistant
    D. The Association of periOperative Registered Nurses Accreditation Guideline

96. To MOST effectively evaluate a patient's comprehension of their upcoming surgery, the nurse will:
    A. Ask the patient to describe the procedure in their own words
    B. Witness the patient signing the consent form
    C. Ask the patient questions about the surgery
    D. Document that the patient has received an educational brochure

97. When forceps are held too tight on the skin, they can create:
    A. Bruises
    B. Scrapes
    C. Burns
    D. Perforations

98. Which of the following situations is an example of a sentinel event?
    A. A patient who received surgery on the wrong body part
    B. A patient who developed a Stage II pressure ulcer during surgery
    C. A patient who received an extra dose of an antibiotic before surgery
    D. A patient who developed a surgical wound infection after surgery

99. The nurse maintains a strict sterile technique while handling surgical supplies and equipment. The nurse's role is:
    A. Circulating nurse
    B. Scrub nurse
    C. First assistant nurse
    D. Advanced practice nurse

100. Proper disposal of infectious, nonhazardous, and hazardous material promotes what type of safety?
    A. Patient safety
    B. Environmental safety
    C. Employee safety
    D. Financial safety

101. The preoperative nurse is providing treatment for a patient when a family member suddenly begins to exhibit aggressive behaviors. What should the nurse do to ensure quality care and promote positive outcomes?
    A. Document all statements (and reactions) made by the patient, staff, and family member
    B. Document findings from the incident in the medical record using an objective manner
    C. Record assumptions, conclusions, and subjective data regarding the family life of the patient
    D. Complete an incident report to reduce the incidence of malpractice suits filed by the family

102. What is the distance recommended for a personal zone?
    A. 0 to 18 inches
    B. 18 inches to 4 feet
    C. 4 to 12 feet
    D. 12 to 25 feet

103. The perioperative nurse has a responsibility to promote environmental best practices by conserving natural resources, reducing waste, and reducing exposure to hazardous materials. What is the BEST way for the nurse to encourage these practices?
    A. Patient education
    B. Physician education
    C. Family education
    D. Team education

104. Which of the following is a true statement regarding the perioperative nurse's role in the informed-consent process?
     A. The nurse is responsible for explaining the procedure to the patient
     B. The nurse is responsible for informing the patient of the risks of the procedure
     C. The nurse is responsible for clarifying information about the procedure as required
     D. The nurse is responsible for signing the informed consent form and acknowledging that the patient understands all required information

105. Which of the following labs indicates the nutritional status of a patient?
     A. Cholesterol
     B. Albumin
     C. Fasting glucose level
     D. Hemoglobin

106. Perioperative RNs should not be required to work for more than how many consecutive hours in a 24-hour period?
     A. 8 hours
     B. 10 hours
     C. 12 hours
     D. 14 hours

107. Which of the following is a human factor that can affect communication during intraoperative care?
     A. Fatigue
     B. Cold room temperature
     C. Background equipment noise
     D. Conversations between the surgeon and surgical technician

108. The nurse can BEST keep a patient's information confidential by:
     A. Providing information on a need-to-know basis
     B. Shredding any information no longer needed
     C. Asking the patient who is allowed to receive information about their care
     D. Requiring a passcode before giving any information

109. The postoperative nurse forgets to obtain intraoperative vitals during hand-off communication. The nurse's MOST appropriate action is to:
     A. Call the intraoperative nurse to obtain the vitals
     B. Take the patient's vitals now
     C. Check the patient's chart for the documented vitals
     D. Ask the patient if they remember their vital signs

110. What does the acronym I PASS the BATON represent in a hand-off communication?
    A. Introduction, patient, allergies, situation, safety concerns, the background, actions, timing, ownership, next
    B. Introduction, patient, assessment, situation, safety concerns, the background, actions, timing, ownership, next
    C. Introduction, procedure, assessment, surgical procedure, safety system, the background, allergies, timing, ownership, next
    D. Information, procedure, assessment, safety system, situation, the background, actions, timing ownership, next

111. In which position should a patient undergoing a radical perineal prostatectomy for prostate cancer be placed?
    A. Prone
    B. High lithotomy
    C. Low lithotomy
    D. Lateral

112. When performing a preoperative assessment on a female patient, the nurse should always inquire about the patient's:
    A. Birth control use
    B. Pregnancy history
    C. Last menstrual cycle
    D. Most recent mammogram results

113. A patient with a body mass index (BMI) of 41 is scheduled for an oophorectomy. The patient has a history of difficult Foley catheter placement. The nurse should:
    A. Inform the surgeon that they will not be able to place the Foley catheter
    B. Place the Foley catheter after the patient is prepped in the OR
    C. Place the Foley catheter preoperatively
    D. Ask the surgeon to insert a suprapubic catheter

114. Interdisciplinary team members in the surgical setting can MOST effectively deliver safe and effective care by exhibiting which of the following characteristics?
    A. Accountability and sustainability
    B. Accountability and reliability
    C. Responsibility and accountability
    D. Responsibility and reliability

115. During the set-up of the OR, the nurse notices that the forceps are hanging over the edge of the sterile field. The surgeon is anxious to get started as they are already 30 minutes behind schedule. The nurse's BEST action is to:
    A. Move the forceps into the sterile field
    B. Extend the sterile field so it encompasses the forceps
    C. Remove all instruments and restart with new sterile instruments
    D. Leave the forceps alone; they are sterile and moving them would break the sterile field

116. What two roles start the surgical count?
    A. Circulating nurse and surgeon
    B. Circulating nurse and scrub nurse
    C. Circulating nurse and nurse anesthetist
    D. Circulating nurse and advanced practice nurse

117. Which of the following is an example of a type-III necrotizing fasciitis?
    A. Aerobic
    B. Anaerobic
    C. Beta-hemolytic streptococcus
    D. Vibrio

118. Which of the following scenarios is MOST concerning regarding gown–glove practice?
    A. When the glove offers no anti-slip properties
    B. When the glove is pulled over the sleeve
    C. When the glove slips down on the sleeve
    D. When the glove rolls down on the sleeve

119. Chemicals that are bioaccumulative and suspected/known carcinogens are:
    A. Air toxins
    B. Waste products
    C. Chemicals of concern
    D. The waste stream

120. Which patient would require more specific preoperative assessment, evaluation, and treatment as a result of their current medication regimen?
    A. A man who regularly takes nonsteroidal anti-inflammatory drugs for his rheumatoid arthritis
    B. A woman who takes a daily thyroid medication for hypothyroidism
    C. A man who takes an angiotensin-converting enzyme inhibitor for chronic hypertension
    D. A woman who takes daily anticoagulants to treat atrial fibrillation

121. A 55-kg patient is experiencing local anesthetic systemic toxicity. The nurse administered amiodarone for their arrhythmia and is now preparing to administer lipid emulsion 20%. After the bolus, the nurse will set the pump to deliver what infusion rate?
    A. 1,815 mL/hr
    B. 600 mL/hr
    C. 1,050 mL/hr
    D. 825 mL/hr

122. Which preoperative practice helps to prevent emergency situations in the OR?
    A. Time-out
    B. Briefing
    C. Preprocedural checklist
    D. Comprehensive surgical checklist

123. Which of the following is one of the three components of an OR fire?
  A. Heat
  B. Combustion
  C. Ignition source
  D. Gas source

124. Which of the following indicates that a patient may be at increased risk for postoperative deep vein thrombosis?
  A. History of varicosities
  B. History of alcohol abuse
  C. Recent upper respiratory infection
  D. Body mass index greater than 26

125. Which of the following is an OR culture that inhibits effective team communication and increases the risk of error?
  A. Lack of knowledge
  B. Lack of credibility
  C. Limited skill set
  D. Feelings of intimidation

126. What areas should the nurse focus on in the preoperative period to promote positive outcomes?
  A. Allergies, pain, fear
  B. Allergies, nutrition, anxiety
  C. Anxiety, pain, nutrition
  D. Anxiety, fear, knowledge

127. During the resuscitation of a patient with local anesthetic systemic toxicity, what is the recommended dosage of epinephrine?
  A. 1,000 mcg
  B. 5,000 mcg
  C. Less than 1 mcg/kg
  D. Greater than 1 mcg/kg

128. Which of the following BEST describes the role of the peri-anesthesia nurse in the transfer of care?
  A. To help the patient return to their baseline
  B. To assist the patient with discharge
  C. To prepare the patient for self-care at home
  D. To assess the patient for complications

129. What type of surgical instrument processing is required for items that have come in direct contact with the vascular system?
  A. Sterilization
  B. Intermediate-level disinfection
  C. Low-level disinfection
  D. Cleaning with sterile saline

130. The postoperative nurse is utilizing the situation, background, assessment, and recommendation (SBAR) method to call a report to the nurse who will be accepting the surgical patient. Which information will the nurse include in the "S" portion?
    A. Required tests
    B. Vital signs
    C. Mental status
    D. Recommendations

131. A postoperative nurse is developing an educational plan for a patient and their wife for postoperative care. What is the MOST important factor to consider when developing a communication method?
    A. The patient's educational level
    B. Their schedule
    C. The patient's relationship with their spouse
    D. Additional support systems

132. The circulating nurse is documenting during surgery. The patient begins to twitch and heart rate increases from 85 bpm to 125 bpm. Which of the following is the MOST accurate statement regarding this patient?
    A. The patient is doing fine, and all vitals are stable
    B. The anesthesia is not adequate, and the dose needs to be adjusted
    C. The patient is having an adverse reaction, and the surgery needs to stop
    D. The patient is experiencing a normal phenomenon that occurs with induction

133. What is the preferred type of needle for subcutaneous suturing?
    A. Blunt
    B. Keith
    C. Reverse cut
    D. Taper cut

134. What is the intraoperative nurse's first priority when caring for a trauma patient?
    A. Maintaining airway
    B. Minimizing pain and blood loss
    C. Starting an IV for rapid fluid infusion
    D. Drawing blood for a type screen and match

135. The nurse is prepping a patient for a left lateral thoracotomy to fix a ventricular septal defect. The patient's left arm is securely strapped to the arm board and abducted 70 degrees from the body. The left arm is abducted at this angle to:
    A. Bring the arm closer to the body to prevent hyperextension of the intercostal spaces
    B. Move the arm away from the body to allow access to the left side intercostal spaces
    C. Move the arm anteriorly to ensure it is out of the surgeon's way
    D. Reduce risk of brachial nerve plexus injury

136. Which psychosocial emotion is most common for a patient during the preoperative phase?
    A. Fear
    B. Anger
    C. Depression
    D. Frustration

137. What intervention should the preoperative nurse use with a patient who has a latex allergy?
    A. Avoid using tubing that has polyvinyl chloride
    B. Apply a cloth barrier to the arm under the blood pressure cuff
    C. Use medications from ampules that have rubber stoppers
    D. Avoid using medications from ampules

138. The surgeon is performing a laparoscopic procedure to better visualize the patient's uterus. The nurse preps the procedure field to include:
    A. Hulka tenaculum
    B. Vise-grip pliers
    C. Curettes
    D. Gouges

139. During pre-admission, a patient asks the nurse if they should proceed with their leg amputation. The nurse's MOST appropriate response is:
    A. "I would if I were you."
    B. "I think you should."
    C. "What do you think you should do?"
    D. "Everyone feels this way before an amputation."

140. The nurse is caring for a patient who is experiencing an acute anaphylactic reaction. The nurse will prepare to administer:
    A. Dantrolene
    B. Epinephrine
    C. Corticosteroids
    D. Hydroxyzine

141. A surgical item with a gauze string attached to one end to secure bulky dressings is a:
    A. Stockinette
    B. Montgomery strap
    C. Nonallergenic tape
    D. Four-ply crinkle gauze

142. The nurse is educating a patient about the use of incentive spirometry (ICS) following surgery. The patient asks the nurse how it helps the lungs after surgery. The nurse's BEST response is:
    A. "ICS minimizes inflation of your lungs and prevents you from having to breathe so deeply."
    B. "ICS minimizes inflation of your lungs and reduces the risk of pneumonia."
    C. "ICS maximizes inflation of your lungs and reduces the risk of pneumonia."
    D. "ICS maximizes inflation of your lungs and completely diminishes the risk of pneumonia."

143. Which cycle should be used when performing immediate-use steam sterilization on a small instrument set that includes a Yankauer suction and a small-powered instrument?
    A. 250 degrees Fahrenheit for 10 minutes
    B. Cycle outlined in manufacturer's instructions for the set and container
    C. 270 degrees Fahrenheit for 4 minutes
    D. Cycle outlined in OSHA standards

144. What is the orientation period for a new perioperative nurse?
    A. 3 to 6 months
    B. 6 to 9 months
    C. 6 to 12 months
    D. 12 to 18 months

145. A patient asks to donate their own blood before a scheduled surgery to prepare for the possibility that they may require a blood transfusion. This is classified as a _____ blood donation.
    A. Direct
    B. Homologous
    C. Heterologous
    D. Autologous

146. When should pressure-injury prevention begin?
    A. During the surgical procedure
    B. Directly after the surgery is completed
    C. Before the patient enters the surgical suite
    D. 24 hours after the surgery

147. The circulating nurse is handing out eye protection to the OR staff. One staff member says they do not need the eye goggles because they have glasses on and that will protect them from laser emissions. The nurse's BEST response is:
    A. "The glasses you are wearing will be sufficient; however, do not remove them."
    B. "The glasses you are wearing are not sufficient."
    C. "If your glasses are tinted, it will be ok."
    D. "Your glasses need to be sterilized before going into the OR."

148. The nurse who is working in the central processing and sterilization area in the surgical setting should follow the guidelines of what organization?
    A. American Society of PeriAnesthesia Nurses
    B. Association for Professionals in Infection Control and Epidemiology
    C. Association for the Advancement of Medical Instrumentation
    D. International Association of Healthcare Central Service Material Management

149. Which of the following is the earliest and most sensitive sign of malignant hyperthermia?
    A. Hypercarbia
    B. Tachycardia
    C. Tachypnea
    D. Muscle rigidity

150. The patient scheduled for amputation has become agitated and irate and refuses surgery. The patient was pleasant earlier and signed consents. The OR has already been set up, and the team has begun to scrub in. The nurse's BEST action is to:
   A. Calm the patient down and inform them the surgery is still happening
   B. Administer a sedative to relax the patient and proceed to the OR
   C. Bring the patient to the OR while explaining that it is too late to cancel
   D. Assess the patient for any physiologic changes and alert the surgical team

151. When are a patient's rights restored after a temporary override?
   A. As soon as possible
   B. When the physician writes the order
   C. 48 hours after the incident
   D. 72 hours after the incident

152. When should decontamination of surgical instruments begin?
   A. One hour prior to the surgical procedure
   B. Immediately upon completion of the surgical procedure
   C. One hour after completion of the surgical procedure
   D. At the point of use during the surgical procedure

153. When does the perioperative nurse ask the patient about any special equipment or implants?
   A. Sign-in
   B. Time-out
   C. Sign-out
   D. Pre-procedure

154. Which of the clinical signs of local anesthetic systemic toxicity would be first according to the classic progression of signs and symptoms?
   A. Confusion
   B. Hypertension
   C. Metallic taste
   D. Respiratory depression

155. Which surgical instrument sterilization method interferes with cell metabolism and the reproduction of the cell?
   A. Ozone gas
   B. Hydrogen peroxide vapor
   C. Ethylene oxide gas
   D. Peracetic acid

156. The nurse is caring for a patient who is being prepped for an appendectomy. The patient's skin tears and bleeds when tape is removed. The nurse alerts the surgeon that the patient:
   A. Needs an occlusive dressing
   B. Has a hypertrophic scar
   C. Has friable skin
   D. Has a wound dehiscence

157. The intraoperative nurse notices the anesthesiologist is about to administer a spinal anesthetic to a patient whose platelet count is 80,000. The nurse will:
    A. Tell the anesthesiologist that what they are doing is wrong
    B. Ask the anesthesiologist why they are administering a spinal anesthetic
    C. Tell the anesthesiologist they are going to kill the patient
    D. Tell the anesthesiologist that administration poses a safety risk

158. What is the minimum number of RN circulators that should be assigned for every patient undergoing a surgical or invasive procedure?
    A. Zero
    B. One
    C. Two
    D. Three

159. Which of the following types of communication can cause miscommunication in the OR?
    A. Formal
    B. Written
    C. Nonverbal
    D. Closed-loop

160. During a preoperative assessment, the nurse is reviewing the patient's current medications. The nurse should document the time of last dose for which of the following drug classes?
    A. Anti-arrhythmias
    B. Angiotensin-converting enzyme inhibitors
    C. Beta blockers
    D. Loop diuretics

161. Which of the following is the MOST accurate statement regarding relative humidity?
    A. Relative humidity can impact the shelf life and product integrity of nonsterile supplies
    B. Relative humidity can impact the shelf life and product integrity of sterile supplies
    C. Relative humidity can impact product integrity of nonsterile supplies
    D. Relative humidity can impact product integrity of sterile supplies

162. Which of the following is an occluding instrument used in surgery?
    A. Scalpel
    B. Hemostat
    C. Forceps
    D. Scissors

163. Which of the following actions MOST effectively promotes patient safety?
    A. Preparing a sterile field
    B. Marking the site for surgery
    C. Reviewing the pre-admission checklist
    D. Ensuring that lighting is adequate for the surgery

164. Which of the following labs, if abnormal, could cause arrhythmias during surgery?
    A. Sodium
    B. Potassium
    C. Hemoglobin
    D. Fasting blood glucose

165. The circulating nurse is talking with a coworker while setting up the OR for the afternoon case. The coworker relays that the patient is very anxious and confided that they take valium multiple times a day to deal with anxiety. The circulating nurse's BEST action is to:
    A. Make a note in the patient's chart
    B. Tell the lead surgeon
    C. Tell the anesthesiologist
    D. Reassure the patient that everything will be fine

166. What type of monitor system is the Bowie-Dick test?
    A. Chemical indicator
    B. Physical monitor
    C. Biologic monitor
    D. Pressure indicator

167. What type of injury is MOST commonly reported by perioperative team members?
    A. Cervical spine
    B. Lumbar spine
    C. Upper extremities
    D. Lower extremities

168. The perioperative nurse manager has called in two surgical nurses due to chronic behavior that is disruptive, unkind, and disrespectful. What is this type of behavior called?
    A. Horizontal violence
    B. Bullying
    C. Abuse
    D. Incivility

169. What preoperative instruction should the nurse provide a patient who takes phenobarbital for seizure prevention?
    A. Do not take it the day of surgery
    B. Continue to take as directed
    C. Discontinue 2 weeks before surgery
    D. Discontinue 24 to 48 hours before surgery

170. Which of the following is a biologic hazard that can occur with the use of lasers?
    A. Plume
    B. Mechanical failure
    C. Electrical shortage
    D. Electrical shock

171. What basic principle of surgical asepsis should the nurse understand when working in the perioperative area?
    A. Isolate any patient who has an infectious disease
    B. Maintain all areas for basic cleanliness
    C. Destroy organisms as they leave the body
    D. Destroy organisms before they enter the body

172. Which of the following is a category used to classify a surgical procedure?
    A. Minor
    B. Radical
    C. Emergent
    D. Diagnostic

173. An experienced nurse is meeting with a novice nurse monthly to provide support, guidance, and advice. The experienced nurse is MOST likely _____ the novice nurse.
    A. Managing
    B. Mentoring
    C. Advocating for
    D. Precepting

174. The acronym SWITCH stands for:
    A. Surgical procedure, wet, instruments, timing, counts, have you any questions
    B. Surgical procedure, wet, instruments, tissue, counts, have you any questions
    C. Sterility, wet, instruments, timing, counts, hand-off
    D. Sterility, wet, instruments, tissues, counts, hand-off

175. Which drug category would the nurse specifically ask about during the assessment of medication use?
    A. Herbal
    B. Prescribed
    C. Psychiatric
    D. Cardiovascular

176. What is the minimum recommended drying time for alcohol-based preps?
    A. 1 minute
    B. 2 minutes
    C. 3 minutes
    D. 5 minutes

177. The nurse is initiating a preoperative assessment and speaks with a patient to obtain information regarding past surgical history. The nurse is engaging in:
    A. Organizational communication
    B. Intrapersonal communication
    C. Interpersonal communication
    D. Group communication

178. Which of the following is the MOST accurate statement regarding efficient inventory management systems?
    A. They improve sterilization procedures
    B. They improve environmental safety
    C. They improve patient outcomes
    D. They improve staffing

179. The patient notes a history of King-Denborough syndrome in their family. While preparing the plan of care, the nurse notes a potential risk for what complication?
    A. Hypoxemia
    B. Malignant hyperthermia
    C. Hypothermia
    D. Anaphylactic reaction

180. The acronym LAST stands for:
    A. Latent anesthetic systemic toxicity
    B. Local anesthetic systemic toxicity
    C. Local anesthetic systemic thrombosis
    D. Latent anesthetic systemic thrombosis

181. The nurse is conducting a preoperative assessment and asks the patient if they have a list of their wishes regarding medical decisions. What is the name of this legal document?
    A. Power of attorney
    B. Healthcare proxy
    C. General will
    D. Advance directive

182. A 34-year-old female patient is undergoing surgery to repair a fractured femur. The patient is 25 weeks' pregnant. What is the appropriate positioning for this patient?
    A. Lateral
    B. Supine
    C. Wedge under left hip
    D. Wedge under right hip

183. Which of the following has the greatest impact on a patient's overall outcomes?
    A. Extent and role of the patient's healthcare provider
    B. Extent and role of the patient's community resources
    C. Extent and role of the patient's support network
    D. Extent and role of the patient's insurance carrier

184. ASRA stands for:
    A. American Society for Regional Anesthesia
    B. American Society of Registered Anesthesiologists
    C. American Society for Registered Anesthesiologists and Surgeons
    D. American Society of Regional Anesthesia and Pain Medicine

185. Which of the following is the MOST accurate statement regarding the storage of sterile items in the intraoperative setting?
     A. Sterile items should be kept in a designated storage room that remains locked
     B. Sterile items should be kept in a double-locked system in a designated area
     C. Sterile items should be stored in covered carts or closed cabinets when outside a sterile room
     D. Sterile items should be kept in a designated sterile room, but they do not need to show an expiration date

186. The nurse is assisting the anesthesiologist with intubation of a patient. The nurse begins to compress the cricoid cartilage before medication administration. The purpose of this maneuver is to:
     A. Occlude the airway so the patient will relax
     B. Occlude the esophagus to allow stabilization
     C. Ensure that the trachea does not move after the patient is sedated
     D. Locate the trachea for the anesthesiologist to promote ease of intubation

187. The pulmonary syndrome that develops following aspiration is influenced by which of the following factors?
     A. Composition of aspirate and length of time since meal
     B. Composition of aspirate and history of acid-reflux disease
     C. Composition of aspirate and history of gastric ulcer
     D. Composition of aspirate and volume of the aspirate

188. Which of the following BEST describes the responsibilities of the scrub nurse?
     A. Educate the patient and family on measures to prevent postoperative complications
     B. Rotate between duties in the preoperative, intraoperative, and postoperative settings
     C. Maintain aseptic conditions and process equipment
     D. Complete a preoperative health assessment and formulate the nursing care plan

189. Which of the following medications is used to treat malignant hyperthermia?
     A. Tizanidine
     B. Dantrolene
     C. Metaxalone
     D. Methocarbamol

190. Which communication technique by the nurse allows the patient to think through a point during the communication process?
     A. Silence
     B. Acceptance
     C. Focusing
     D. Reflecting

191. The nurse is interviewing a patient who starts to talk about her fears regarding surgery. The nurse says, "I am sure everything will be fine. You really have nothing to worry about." The nurse is:
    A. Giving advice
    B. Changing the subject
    C. Being judgmental
    D. Speaking in clichés

192. Which of the following is a patient-dependent fuel source in OR fires?
    A. Hydrogen
    B. Acetone
    C. Benzoin
    D. Ether

193. The patient expresses fear of "being put to sleep." The nurse explains to the patient that they do not need to be concerned because they will be awake during their procedure. Which anesthetic will be used?
    A. General anesthesia
    B. Regional anesthesia
    C. Local anesthesia
    D. Intravenous anesthesia

194. What are two questions included in the surgical time-out?
    A. Correct site? Correct equipment?
    B. Correct location? Correct images?
    C. Correct patient? Correct staff?
    D. Correct procedure? Correct operating room?

195. Which patient is MOST vulnerable to local anesthetic systemic toxicity if lidocaine is used?
    A. Patient with severe liver disease
    B. Patient with respiratory acidosis
    C. Patient with ischemic heart disease
    D. Patient with end-stage renal disease

196. The nurse is assessing a patient and suspects anaphylaxis. Which of the following symptoms led the nurse to this suspicion?
    A. Hypotension and bradycardia
    B. Hypertension and tachycardia
    C. Hypotension and bronchospasm
    D. Bronchospasm and hypertension

197. Which of the following organizations accredits healthcare facilities?
    A. Centers for Medicare and Medicaid Services
    B. Occupational Safety and Health Administration
    C. The Joint Commission
    D. Centers for Disease Control and Prevention

198. In which phase of the standards established by the American Society of PeriAnesthesia Nurses is a patient ready for discharge?
A. Phase I
B. Phase II
C. Phase III
D. Phase IV

199. Once a patient is brought into the OR, the circulating nurse is responsible for:
A. Attending to the patient's needs and performing a review of body systems
B. Marking the correct surgical site with their initials
C. Preparing the OR while the scrub person tends to the patient
D. Directing the entire team's attention to the patient

200. Which procedure has the highest rate of postoperative respiratory failure?
A. Craniotomy
B. Cholecystectomy
C. Femoral-popliteal bypass
D. Abdominal aortic aneurysm repair

1. **B) The follow-up phone call**
   The direct perioperative nurse–patient relationship is terminated at the postoperative assessment or follow-up phone call. The nurse–patient relationship remains after surgery and at all phases of the post-anesthesia care unit (PACU).

2. **C) Sharps container**
   A sharps container should be used to dispose of any item that could stick, cut, or scrape a patient or healthcare worker. It is also an appropriate container for hazardous body fluids. A sharps container is a puncture-proof and leak-proof container and will have the international symbol for biohazard waste on the outside. A biohazard bag would not be appropriate due to the potential injury that could be caused by these hazardous items. A non-biohazard bag or container would not be appropriate for these items because they are all considered to be hazardous materials.

3. **A) Social talk**
   Evidence shows that social talk that is irrelevant conversation can be distracting and interfere with patient-related tasks. This can negatively impact patient outcomes. Communication that is structured, standardized, and closed-loop are facilitators of effective intraoperative communication.

4. **C) Address risk factors that might delay recovery**
   The preoperative period is used to determine the patient's health status; therefore, all assessments conducted during this period address risk factors that may contribute to postoperative complications and delay recovery. Determining the patient's goals for surgery and ensuring necessary checklists are completed are included in the assessment; however, these are not the overall goals of the preoperative assessment. Diagnostic tests are typically completed in the preadmission phase, which proceeds the preoperative phase.

5. **A) Myoglobinuria**
   Malignant hyperthermia (MH) is a severe adverse reaction to anesthetic agents. Myoglobinuria and seizures are late signs of hyperthermia. Early signs of MH include tachycardia, tachypnea, and muscle rigidity.

6. **C) Minimizing overtime use and allowing recuperation time between work hours**

   The Association of periOperative Registered Nurses' (AORN)'s position statement on Perioperative Safe Staffing and On-Call Practices was developed to promote the overall goal of providing a safe, healthy environment for the interdisciplinary team. An adequate staffing schedule provides the personnel needed to work with the patients scheduled for certain surgical and invasive procedures on any given day. An on-call staffing plan is necessary for any unplanned procedure for which the appropriate personnel may not be at the surgical facility, and other team members need to be called in to assist the patient and the surgical team. An adequate on-call staffing plan can work to minimize overtime while allowing staff members to have time between a certain amount of work hours to rest and recuperate. This could help to prevent burnout among the team members and maximize retention of the perioperative RNs on the interdisciplinary team. An unhealthy work environment could develop if extended work hours and overtime are utilized.

7. **B) 10 to 20 minutes**

   Specimens for frozen sections are typically processed within 10 to 20 minutes and are never placed in formalin or a fixative for processing. These could cause the cells in the specimen to be damaged and not be viable for processing. Biopsy specimens are taken (within 10 to 20 minutes) directly to the pathology department by personnel from the intraoperative area. Some facilities have policies that require that an employee from pathology come to the surgical area to collect the specimen.

8. **D) Cutting off circulation in the lower extremities**

   Placing a patient in supine position with legs uncrossed prevents circulation issues in the lower extremities and promotes hemodynamic stability. If the patient is at risk for skin breakdown, a gel pillow can be placed at pressure points. To promote comfort and relieve pressure from the lower back, the nurse can place a wedge underneath the patient's knees. Surgical drapes should cover the patient and table; they do not need to be even.

9. **A) Patient identification, operative consent, allergies**

   The nurse must verify that the right patient is receiving the right surgery and that they have consented to it. Patient identification, operative consent, and allergies are all essential components of the patient's preoperative checklist for surgery. Patient identification typically includes their name, date of birth, and hospital number. Allergy information is important for patient safety. Address and lab results are not part of the preoperative checklist, nor are assigned room and family contact information. Insurance information is not relevant to surgery.

10. **B) Ask the patient in a frank, direct manner.**

    Health history questions addressing illicit drug use should be asked in a frank, direct manner. The nurse should employ a patient and nonjudgmental manner. The nurse should not direct health history questions to a patient's family member as it violates patient privacy. While a questionnaire could be useful, many people who use or abuse drugs often deny use or attempt to hide it. The nurse should never assume anything concerning a patient's health history and should ask all appropriate questions.

11. **D) National Fire Protection Association**
The National Fire Protection Association provides standards for the reduction of hazards and possible exposure to noxious stimuli. The National Quality Forum provides documentation and data on adverse events from medical/surgical errors, personnel errors, and environmental hazards. The American National Standards Institute provides information about exposure to toxic materials. The Centers for Disease Control and Prevention develops and applies disease prevention and control, environmental health, and health promotion and health education activities.

12. **C) "We are not trained to move the anesthesia equipment. Only the anesthesiologist can do that."**
Scrub persons and circulating nurses are not trained to move anesthesia equipment or check the connections. The equipment should be moved only by the anesthesiologist. The anesthesia machine can be moved as soon as the bed is in the proper position; it does not need to be moved last. The equipment in the room can be moved as needed to accommodate the patient and the anesthesiologist.

13. **C) 56%**
Association of periOperative Registered Nurses (AORN) data suggests that supply costs can make up at least 56% of the total operating room budget. AORN provides recommendations for how the perioperative interdisciplinary team can conserve natural resources, reduce waste, and reduce exposure to hazardous materials.

14. **B) Latex products**
Patients with a history of allergic reactions to banana, kiwi, avocado, passion fruit, and chestnuts are at an increased risk for allergy to latex. Latex is made from the milky fluid of rubber tree plants. Latex is a material used in many products in medical and perioperative settings, including gloves, catheter tubing, and medication vials. Allergic reactions to antimicrobial infusions, corticosteroid injections, and metal instruments are not associated with banana and kiwi allergies.

15. **C) Full Code**
During surgery, all patients are Full Code. The patient would not be returned to his do not intubate (DNI) status until after surgery. DNR is do not resuscitate, which the patient did not indicate. A DNR/DNI is indicated for a patient who does not want to be resuscitated or intubated.

16. **B) Negative**
Negative airflow will pull ambient air out of the room, which is required when decontaminating and sterilizing equipment. Positive airflow pulls air and airborne particles into the room, which can potentially contaminate the equipment.

17. **A) Mentor**
The experienced perioperative nurse is practicing the role of mentor. This strategy works by providing the novice nurse with the opportunity to work with an experienced nurse in a specific specialty area, for as long as needed, to gain knowledge and skills for patient care. A preceptorship is considered a more short-term assignment and consists of a set number of hours and/or days. The role of advocate is to

promote and support an individual, organization, or group by speaking up on their behalf and does not involve teaching knowledge and skills to novice nurses. A manager would be part of the leadership team that would promote a mentorship between the experienced nurse and the novice nurse. The manager could possibly be the one who matches the two nurses together.

18. **B) Control the spread of infection**
Terminal cleaning is used in the surgical setting to control the spread of infection. It is an extensive cleaning process in which every item in the surgical room is detached and disinfected, including light fixtures and air vents. The walls and ceiling are also cleaned. Terminal cleaning must be completed prior to accepting surgical patients back into the surgical suite. It does not control air particle exposure. Healthcare personnel must wear a mask, and possibly a face shield or N95 mask, depending on the particles that will be dispensed during the disinfectant process. Controlling the use of disinfectants and sterilization is not the purpose of terminal cleaning.

19. **C) Administer lipid emulsion**
The patient in this scenario is experiencing signs of severe local anesthetic systemic toxicity (LAST) and requires lipid emulsion therapy. Propofol should not be used because it has low lipid content and has direct cardiac depressant effects. Lorazepam may be used to increase the seizure threshold, but would be considered after the patient has recovered. If the patient remains hypotensive after recovery, norepinephrine bitartrate may be considered to increase blood pressure.

20. **A) Close to three quarters**
The Association of periOperative Registered Nurses (AORN) position statement notes that the perioperative setting of a facility generates approximately 70% of the total waste. It is also estimated that the perioperative area can consume three to six times more energy per square foot than other areas of the hospital.

21. **C) Class III**
A verified appendicitis means that an active infection has been identified. Class III wounds are known to be contaminated. Open wounds that are fresh and caused from a major break in sterile technique and leakage into the wound also fall into this category, as do open traumatic wounds that are more than 12 to 24 hours old. An uninfected operative wound is a Class I (clean) wound. Class II (clean contaminated) wounds are exposed to various tracts of the body without unusual contamination. Class IV (dirty) wounds display obvious infection with pus.

22. **C) Administer 100% oxygen**
The patient is exhibiting symptoms of postoperative anaphylaxis. Anaphylaxis reactions cause severe respiratory distress. The nurse's best initial action is to administer oxygen at 100% and maintain a patent airway. After the patient is stabilized, the nurse would notify the anesthesiologist for further orders. These orders may include fluids to maintain fluid balance and the administration of corticosteroids to help prevent or control a late-phase reaction, which could take up to 36 hours to manifest.

23. A) Excretion ability

The kidneys excrete drugs and waste products. Patients who have kidney or urinary impairments have decreased ability to excrete drugs and anesthetic agents, which can impact drug effectiveness and increase the risk for toxicity. Preoperative assessment of a patient's kidney function does not determine their tolerance for a urinary catheter or whether an infection is present. When assessing kidney function, the nurse may ask questions related to the patient's ability to urinate independently, but it is not the primary reason for performing the assessment.

24. D) Surgical site infection

Delayed wound healing among patients undergoing a surgical or other invasive procedure is most often linked to surgical site infections (SSIs), which typically occur within 30 days of the procedure. Immunocompromised status, diabetes, and smoking can all increase risk for developing a surgical site infection but are not the most common causes.

25. D) Single-use device

The Association of periOperative Registered Nurses (AORN) position statement regarding environmental responsibility of the perioperative nurse recommends several ways to reduce waste, including the reprocessing of single-use medical equipment and devices according to guidelines developed by the U.S. Food and Drug Administration (FDA). A double-use device would not be recommended due to an increased risk for contamination and for potential breakdown of the device after several reprocessing cycles. An implant would not be reprocessed after the initial use due to an increased risk of contamination. If an implant must be removed, it would be discarded per the policy and procedure of the surgical facility.

26. B) Stop the flow of all airway gases

When a fire breaks out in the OR, the first priority is to stop the flow of all airway gases, which are oxidizers. The patient should then be removed from the OR. It may be difficult to identify the source of the fire, so time should not be wasted trying to ascertain the cause. Fires must be extinguished by a specific class of extinguishers; blankets should not be used.

27. A) Powerlessness

The patient's statement indicates that he believes he has lost power by not having the ability to walk independently. Ineffective coping is not appropriate at this time because it is too early to determine if the patient will recover effectively after the surgery. Anticipatory grieving is common among surgical patients, but the patient's statement speaks more to them losing independence and power as a result of their limb amputation. The belief is present and not anticipated. The patient is at risk for disturbed body image, but their statement presents an actual problem, not a risk.

28. B) Tryptase level

Tryptase concentration levels are a highly sensitive marker for diagnosing anaphylaxis. Histamine is not an adequate diagnostic marker because it may be immediately elevated, but may return to baseline during resuscitation. The intradermal test (IDT) and skin prick test (SPT) are used to determine the cause of the anaphylactic reaction. They are typically completed 4 to 6 weeks postreaction.

29. C) Leave the towel where it is and place a new sterile towel over it

The nurse should implement the "place it once" principle from the 8Ps of OR set up. The blood-soaked towel should stay where it is, and a new sterile towel should be placed over it. The nurse should take care to not cover any tools still required. The towel should not be removed as it increases risk that instruments may fall out of the sterile field. The nurse should not obtain a new Mayo stand as this would break the sterile field. It is not necessary in this situation.

30. C) Policy

The nurse who is working to improve healthcare at local, state, and national levels is advocating for changes in policy. The American Nurses Advocacy Institute (ANAI) was developed in 2009 to inspire nurses to become stronger leaders in politics and to motivate the development and maintenance of policy change within local, state, and national levels of government. The program focuses on legislative and regulatory priorities, the advancement of policy issues, and the education of political issues.

31. A) Contact the surgeon to hold the surgery

The potassium level of 2.0 is very low and could cause arrhythmias during surgery. The level must be corrected before the patient can undergo surgery. The nurse's best action is to contact the surgeon so the surgery can be placed on hold. Starting 0.9% of NaCl will not address the potassium level and may in fact cause it to decrease even lower. The fasting glucose level of 95 mg/dL is within normal range, and D50 is not warranted. The nurse would document the labs on the surgical checklist, but the patient should not be sent to surgery prior to correcting the potassium level.

32. B) Minimal exposure to perioperative patient care in nursing curriculum

Most nursing schools provide minimal exposure to the nurse in a perioperative setting in basic nursing curriculum. There is very little time in nursing school for instructors to focus on a nursing role in specialty areas, such as the operating room (OR). The minimal exposure is not due to a lack of interest on the part of the nursing instructors or a lack of interest on the part of the surgical management team. The nursing jobs in this specialty area favor a mentorship-type program that includes a hands-on approach for education and training.

33. B) Virchow's Triad

Venous thromboembolism (VTE) usually occurs from a deep vein thrombosis (DVT) in the lower extremities. Patients with VTE exhibit Virchow's triad: Damage to the vessel, venous stasis, and hypercoagulability. Charcot's triad—fever with rigors, right upper quadrant abdominal pain, and jaundice—is seen in patients with ascending cholangitis. Beck's triad—muffled heart sounds, jugular venous distention, and hypotension—is seen in patients with cardiac tamponade. Cushing's triad—bradycardia, irregular respirations, and hypertension—is seen in patients with intracranial pressure.

34. C) Head covering, face shield, long-cuffed utility gloves, gown, shoe covers

The Association of periOperative Registered Nurses (AORN) recommends the following personal protective equipment (PPE) in the decontamination area: Head covering, face shield, long-cuffed utility gloves, gown, and shoe covers. These PPE items protect the nurse from exposure to contaminated materials. A mask and goggles would not provide sufficient facial covering. Studies have shown that one pair of long-cuffed utility gloves provides the necessary protection against contamination; two pairs of regular gloves are not required.

35. B) Penrose drain

A Penrose drain is a thin radiopaque latex drain that is inserted during surgery to promote drainage of the wound during the postop period. A Foley catheter is a sterile rubber drain used to capture constant urinary drainage. A hemovac is a closed-wound suction device that offers suction postsurgery. It is typically sterile plastic. A Jackson Pratt is another type of plastic drainage reservoir used to promote a closed-suction system.

36. A) Repeat it back before hanging up

Telephones are permissible. All telephone orders require a read-back to ensure accuracy of the order and must be documented. It is the nurse's responsibility to write the order either by hand or in electronic form before carrying out the order. The nurse, not the pharmacist, is responsible for clarifying the accuracy of the order.

37. A) Disaster recall

Disaster recall is the notification of critical staff members needed to report to the facility to participate in patient care. The filtration zone is the area where the patients from the affected area seek assistance. Reverse triage is the process in which space is cleared to make room for patients affected by the disaster, including discharging stable patients, transferring less-critical patients to other hospitals, and canceling elective surgeries. Surge capacity is the process by which healthcare facilities and the surrounding community manage a large influx of patients due to accidents, natural disasters, and terrorist attacks.

38. B) To hold all communications in strict confidentiality

It is most critical for the nurse to remember that all information should be held in strict confidentiality according to the Health Insurance Portability and Accountability Act (HIPAA) regulations. Although it is important to clarify information stated by the patient, document their answers, and ask difficult questions in a direct and frank manner, they are not the most critical considerations in this scenario.

39. B) Electrocautery ablation and laser ablation

The most common surgical smoke-producing procedures used in surgery are electrocautery ablation and laser ablation. Ablation is the removal of unhealthy tissue from the body, which can be performed during surgery, or through the use of hormones, drugs, radiofrequency, heat, or extreme cold. Electrocautery ablation uses an electric current to heat and remove unhealthy tissue, and laser ablation uses light and heat. Radiation ablation is the process of emitting energy in the form of waves or particles to remove tissue, thus producing no surgical smoke. Rather than use heat, cryoablation uses extreme cold to remove unhealthy tissue.

40. C) Cognitive

The use of imagery, distraction, and self-recitation are examples of cognitive coping strategies. The perioperative nurse should educate patients on ways to decrease anxiety and fear, which can help to reduce postoperative complications and promote physical and psychologic healing. *Affective* is a learning domain that focuses on emotions, perceptions, and interests. *Psychomotor* domain would include a demonstration of a learned skill for teaching. *Physical* domain would show a physical finding to know learning had been met.

41. C) Ventricular tachycardia

The patient is experiencing ventricular tachycardia (V-tach), which is characterized by three or more ventricular beats in a row, at a rate of more than 100 beats a minute. In sinus tachycardia, the sinus node fires between 100 and 180 bpm. Ventricular fibrillation is characterized by rapid, erratic electrical impulses at a rate of 150 to 500 bpm. Pulseless electrical activity (PEA), electromechanical dissociation, is a condition in which the patient has sufficient electrical discharge, but is unresponsive with an impalpable pulse.

42. B) A do not resuscitate

When a patient expresses a desire to not be resuscitated, the healthcare provider must give an order for DNR (do not resuscitate). It would need to be documented in all areas so healthcare personnel know the status for the patient. If a DNR order is not given and/or documented, the patient would legally need to be resuscitated, which would go against their current wishes. There does not necessarily need to be an order that the patient is cleared for surgery, unless a problem occurred with testing or informed consent prior to the procedure. The surgery would not be canceled or postponed due to the DNR decision of the patient.

43. A) World Health Organization and Centers for Disease Control and Prevention

Healthcare-associated infections (HAIs) are a patient safety issue affecting all types of healthcare facilities. According to the Centers for Disease Control and Prevention (CDC), millions of patients acquire an infection while receiving care, treatment, and services in a medical facility. Effective hand hygiene is one of the most important ways to address HAIs. Improving compliance with the World Health Organization (WHO) or the CDC hand hygiene guidelines will reduce the transmission of infectious agents by staff to patients, thereby decreasing the incidence of HAIs. The healthcare facility needs to follow only one of the two organizational guidelines. The Centers for Medicare and Medicaid Services (CMS) is a federal health insurance program for individuals aged 65 years or older. The Joint Commission (TJC) surveys hospital facilities for accreditation, but they have not developed specific guidelines for hand hygiene.

44. C) "What do you know about debriefing?"

The nurse should use the same techniques that would be used when educating a patient. First, the nurse must establish a baseline of what the new nurse knows about debriefing to inform what information the nurse should provide. Inquiring about perioperative experience and how long the nurse has been out of school may help the experienced nurse determine the level in which the information should be communicated, but is not the most appropriate response. Nor is simply telling the nurse where they can access information on debriefing.

45. A) Tourniquet

Hemostasis is the act of restricting or stopping blood flow from a damaged vessel or organ. Hemostasis can be induced with chemical, thermal, and mechanical means. A tourniquet is an example of mechanical hemostasis. Fibrin glue is an example of chemical hemostasis. Electrosurgery units and lasers are examples of thermal hemostasis.

46. **B. Dantrolene**
In this scenario, the patient has malignant hyperthermia (MH). Dantrolene, a muscle relaxer, is the first line of treatment for this condition. Dantrolene has been shown to significantly decrease the mortality rate of MH. Tizanidine, metaxalone, and methocarbamol are all muscle relaxers, but they are not used for the treatment of MH.

47. **A) Remove the propofol**
The patient is experiencing severe local anesthetic systemic toxicity (LAST). The nurse should remove the propofol because it has low lipid content and direct cardiac depressant effects. After it is removed, a lipid emulsion should be started. Lorazepam may be used to increase the seizure threshold, but would be considered after the patient has recovered. If the patient remains hypotensive after recovery, norepinephrine bitartrate may be considered to increase blood pressure.

48. **D) "The catheter is inserted during surgery, so you won't feel it."**
Anxiety is common in preoperative holding. A pediatric patient with worries about a catheter or any other aspect of surgery should be provided with an honest but reassuring explanation of what to expect. Belittling or dismissing the anxiety is not appropriate.

49. **D) Disseminated intravascular coagulation**
Disseminated intravascular coagulation (DIC) occurs when coagulation is diffusely activated, causing the development of microthrombi in smaller blood vessels, as well as coagulation factor consumption. The primary trigger is systemic inflammation following traumatic injury. Rhabdomyolysis is muscle damage and cell destruction that results from the release of a muscle protein called myoglobin into the circulation. This process compromises blood flow to the renal system. Hemorrhage occurs when blood vessels rupture or are severed due to trauma. Hypoxemia occurs when levels of oxygen in the blood are lower than normal.

50. **D) Mathematical expression of the probability that an organism is present on an item after sterilization**
The sterility assurance level is a mathematical expression of the probability that an organism is still present on an item after completion of the sterilization process. Thermal death time is the mathematical expression of the time and level of temperature needed to kill microorganisms. A biologic indicator provides information on whether necessary conditions were met to kill a specified number of microorganisms during a given sterilization process.

51. **A) American Society of PeriAnesthesia Nurses**
The American Society of PeriAnesthesia Nurses (ASPAN) has issued standards and guidelines for perianesthesia. It includes position statements, recommendations for practice in perianesthesia, and updated resources from other organizations that partner with ASPAN. The Association for the Advancement of Medical Instrumentation (AAMI) develops standards for enhancing the safety, efficacy, safe use, and management of medical devices and health technologies. The International Association of Healthcare Central Service Material Management (IAHCSMM) supports sterile processing and related professionals. The Association for Professionals in Infection Control and Epidemiology (APIC) is a member organization for infection preventionists.

52. A) Accent

A perioperative team member with an accent can be a barrier for effective communication among the team. Depending on the accent, it may be difficult to understand what the team member is saying and can increase frustration among the team and inhibit positive communication. Time pressure, emotional stress, and multitasking are all considered environmental factors that inhibit effective perioperative communication.

53. C) Release of gaseous byproducts into the atmosphere

The heat from a diathermy causes the rupture of cell membranes, which causes a plume of smoke to develop. This generates a plume of smoke containing mostly water vapor which releases into the atmosphere of the operating room. While surgical smoke is not considered to be an immediate danger, the health concern is due to the different types of contaminants that surgical smoke contains, including contagious, viable malignant cells; live bacteria; and viruses (which could involve human papilloma-virus [HPV], HIV, etc.). "Surgical smoke" is a term used for gaseous byproducts that are produced via energy-productive surgical instruments. The diathermy does not cause release of gaseous byproducts into the body tissue, surgical instrument, or back into the patient, but instead releases it into the atmo-sphere of the operating room. This causes potential harm to the healthcare personnel working in the intraoperative setting.

54. B) Patient Bill of Rights

The basic rule of conduct that exists between patients and the members of a healthcare team is the Patient Bill of Rights. It is a general statement that promotes patient confidentiality and dignity, access to care, and consent to treatment and is adopted by most healthcare facilities. The Code of Ethics is comprised of formal guidelines developed by the American Nurses Association that address ethical responsibility and accountability of the nurse. Informed consent is a process of communication between the patient and healthcare provider that provides agreement and permission for care, treatment, or ser-vices. Consumer rights and protections are an element of the Affordable Care Act (ACA). These rights and protections were developed to make healthcare coverage more equitable and easy to understand.

55. B) Be limited to emergency situations

The Centers for Medicare and Medicaid Services (CMS) guidelines state that verbal orders should be limited to emergency situations only. The order must be signed within 48 hours by the provider who gave the order and should be documented by the nurse immediately after taking the order.

56. B) SBAR form

The situation, background, assessment, and recommendation (SBAR) form provides standardized com-munication during the perioperative period among caregivers, including information about the patient during each phase preceding the transfer. Electronic health records (EHR) are charts used for recording patients' care. Although it may be used to obtain patient information, some healthcare facilities' health records are not standardized between units and can lead to fragmented or missing information. The surgical safety checklist was developed to promote effective communication specific for the surgical setting to reduce errors. An incident report is used in all areas of healthcare to identify safety hazards. It is not specific to surgical patient care and safety.

57. D) Bachelor's degree in nursing

Effective January 1, 2020, the education level for entry into the RN first assistant (RNFA) profession is the bachelor's degree. The associate degree and diploma degree would not be considered a sufficient entry level degree for the RNFA.

58. B) Muscle will be separated along fascial layers

Splitting occurs when the surgeon separates muscles along the layer of the fascia during the surgery. Removing blood and fluid from the surgical site is suctioning. Displacing structures with an instrument is retraction. Stopping the flow of blood is hemostasis.

59. B) Adverse metabolic reactions to anesthesia

Adverse metabolic reactions to anesthesia (AMRA) is an acronym used by the Malignant Hyperthermia Association of the United States. AMRA is a form that is completed by an anesthesiologist or another healthcare provider after a patient experiences an adverse metabolic/muscular reaction to anesthesia. The AMRA form is the official documentation of the incident.

60. A) Penicillin

Penicillin is the most common cause of anaphylaxis and accounts for approximately 75% of fatal anaphylactic reactions in the United States. Although patients may be allergic to ciprofloxacin, clindamycin, and metronidazole, and even experience anaphylaxis, they are not the most common cause.

61. D) Local anesthetic system toxicity

The symptoms surfaced after administration of local anesthetic, so the patient is likely experiencing local anesthetic system toxicity (LAST). This is the central nervous system's response to the toxic effects of a local anesthetic. During a syncope episode, a patient may experience lightheadedness but not tinnitus and blurred vision. The lightheadedness is a result of a fall in blood pressure. Meniere's disease's hallmark symptom is tinnitus, but it is absent of the blurred vision and has no relationship to receiving a local anesthetic. Hypotension can cause a patient to be lightheaded, but orthostatic hypotension occurs when a patient stands and their blood pressure drops.

62. A) Dissection

Dissection is the act of separating the tissue from muscles/skin/organ during a surgical procedure. There are both sharp and blunt methods to dissection. Harvesting is the removal of an organ for the purpose of transplantation. Traction is force applied to the skin so that it remains taught. Procurement is the act of obtaining an object, such as obtaining a valve for replacement.

63. A) Aspiration

The risk of aspiration occurs more frequently during the initiation of anesthetic drugs. Rapid sequence induction is an algorithm utilized to decrease the risk of aspiration in high-risk patients by protecting the patient's airway. This process was developed for use in emergency surgeries and high-risk patients to reduce the risk of aspiration of stomach contents into the lung. Pulmonary aspiration of regurgitated stomach contents is an emergent situation due to the pulmonary conditions it can produce. Pulmonary edema can occur when excessive fluids and blood products are administered to a patient who is hemorrhaging during surgery. Laryngospasm involves a spasm of the vocal cords that can cause temporary difficulty in breathing for the patient. Hemorrhage can happen suddenly during surgery if a blood vessel ruptures or is accidentally severed or if the patient has suffered some type of trauma.

64. D) Caffeine-halothane contracture test

The gold standard test for diagnosing malignant hyperthermia (MH) is the caffeine-halothane contracture test (CHCT). It has 9% sensitivity and 78% specificity. The in vitro contracture test is the European counterpart. Genetic testing and DNA sampling can be completed to diagnose MH, but they are not the gold standard tests.

65. B) Notify the surgeon

The RN circulator should inform and receive verbal acknowledgement from the surgeon and surgical team as soon as a discrepancy in a surgical count is identified. The next likely action is to repeat the count. If the count remains incorrect, the supervisor should be notified, and an x-ray obtained. If the count continues to be incorrect, the discrepancy should be documented.

66. C) Circulating nurse

Fuel sources that contribute to operating fires are usually supplied by the circulating nurse or scrub technician, including sponges, drapes, and other flammable items. The anesthesiologist usually supplies the oxidizers, and the surgeon and RN first assistant usually supply the ignition.

67. A) Previous reactions will guide the medication selection for this surgery.

There are multiple factors to be considered when initiating anesthesia. The nurse should always ask the patient about previous anesthesia use and any associated reactions. This will guide the anesthesiologist in selecting the appropriate medication to avoid adverse side effects. The reactions do need to be charted, and it is a matter of protocol, but these answers do not provide rationale for why the information needs to be obtained.

68. C) Discontinue triggering agents

The first response of the surgical team should be to discontinue the triggering agent to prevent further damage. The team would then hyperventilate with 100% oxygen, followed by the administration of a skeletal muscle relaxant and sodium bicarbonate to treat acidosis, which may occur.

69. B) While sutures can be flipped into the sterile field, implants should never be flipped.

Flipping items into the sterile field is a common practice by circulating nurses, since they are not a sterile team member and cannot fully handle sterile supplies. Sutures and other small, rigid items may be flipped into the sterile field with caution. Larger items such as implants should never be flipped into the sterile field as it increases risk for contamination or accidently flipping them onto the floor. The sterile field should not be enlarged to accommodate flipped items.

70. C) Open-ended

An open-ended questioning method should be employed to allow the patient the opportunity to give as much information as they can according to their comfort level. Direct and closed-ended methods could lead to information being left out because the patient is answering only the questions asked. A probing questioning method may seem intrusive and could lead to the patient not being forthcoming.

71. A) Surgical comfort vs. risks related to patient position

Inadequate or improper patient positioning in the perioperative area can lead to negative patient outcomes. Patient positioning in the perioperative setting should begin during the preoperative evaluation and continue throughout all phases of the surgical experience. A nurse should promote ideal patient positioning, which involves balancing surgical comfort against the risks related to the patient position. Potential medical consequences related to improper or inadequate positioning include respiratory problems, circulatory problems, pressure ulcers and other skin problems, and neurologic problems. These problems can occur within a few minutes so education should be reinforced to ensure proper patient positioning in the perioperative setting. Patient safety should be a goal for any nurse in any setting. Knowledge of surgical procedure and number of surgical team members needed for a specific procedure is not used to determine ideal positioning.

72. A) Hyperkalemia

Hyperkalemia, increased potassium, can increase the risk of cardiac arrest. Hypokalemia is the opposite of hyperkalemia and refers to low levels of potassium in the blood and does not increase the risk of cardiac arrest. Hypermagnesemia refers to an elevated amount of magnesium in the blood, which can be caused by renal failure or in a patient with poor kidney function. Hypomagnesemia refers to a low magnesium concentration and can be caused by inadequate intake of magnesium. It can also be caused by increased absorption or increased excretion due to hypercalcemia. It is not associated with increased risk of cardiac arrest.

73. C) Mental status

The "S" in SBAR stands for situation, which includes vital signs. The "B" stands for background, which includes information about the patient's mental status, skin condition, and oxygen status. The "A" stands for assessment, which includes current physical findings. The "R" stands for recommendations, which includes physician recommendations and required tests.

74. A) When the patient recovers

The evaluation of the degree of attainment of expected outcomes completes the perioperative nursing process. Evaluation can be collected through assessment of the patient postoperatively and through recovery, which completes the nursing process. When a patient is in the post-anesthesia care unit (PACU) and the operating room, they are still in the perioperative period.

75. **C) Ask the nurse to have another nurse relieve them of their duties.**

A nurse who is yawning is exhibiting signs of fatigue. Fatigue can affect communication and performance in the OR. The nurse should be relieved by another nurse who is rested and able to perform the tasks safely and efficiently. The surgical schedule is made to accommodate the surgeon and patient and should be rescheduled only by unexpected and unavoidable events. Giving the nurse coffee is not the most effective way to handle this situation, for there is no guarantee that it would be effective. Decreasing the temperature within the room may make other team members uncomfortable and does not address the fatigue of the circulating nurse.

76. **B) Place the patient in reverse Trendelenburg position**

The circulating nurse should be familiar with different positions used in the OR and their intended effects. To decrease intracranial pressure, the patient should be placed in reverse Trendelenburg position. Trendelenburg position would increase intracranial pressure. Supine is the standard position used in abdominal surgeries, so the patient would already be in this position. Prone position, placing the patient on their stomach, would be inappropriate for abdominal repair surgery.

77. **D) Flexible laryngoscope**

A patient with a body mass index (BMI) of 32 is obese. Obesity increases the risk of a patient developing a difficult airway. The OR should have equipment to manage any type of emergency airway situation, including tracheal intubation, cricothyrotomy, and tracheotomy. A flexible laryngoscope may need to be used in an obese patient. Ice packs, cooling blankets, and dantrolene are measures used in the treatment of a patient with malignant hyperthermia. They would be available in the OR as a matter of course, not because of the patient's BMI data. Mannitol is a diuretic used to decrease swelling and pressure around the brain or inside the eye. It can also be used in acute kidney failure to help with urine production. It is not related to obesity.

78. **C) Scope of practice**

Nurses can delegate certain tasks to unlicensed assistive personnel (UAPs) according to the scope of practice outlined by the Nurse Practice Act in their state of licensure. A nurse can delegate at any time help is required; however, they may do so only if the task is appropriate for the skill level of the UAP. The nurse remains responsible and accountable for the actions of the UAP. Asking another employee to perform a task that is above their skill level, or agreeing to do a task that is outside one's scope of practice, can lead to disciplinary action by the relevant board of nursing. Medicare guidelines are not related to the delegation of tasks to UAPs. Medicare is the federal health insurance program for individuals who are 65 years old and older. The Patient Bill of Rights is a list of guarantees for those receiving medical care. A licensure compact allows a nurse to have a multistate license in their home state and other states that participate in the licensure compact.

79. **D) 7 to 10 days**

Aspirin use should be discontinued a minimum of 7 to 10 days prior to surgery to decrease the risk of postoperative bleeding. It generally takes platelets approximately 10 days to regenerate; therefore, a period of 24 to 48 hours or 3 to 4 days is not long enough to effectively prevent bleeding.

80. **D) You should use it 10 times and repeat every hour when you are awake.**

    Patient education on the use of an incentive spirometer includes explaining that the patient should perform the procedure 10 times, back-to-back, and repeat every hour while the patient is awake. IS should not be used around the clock.

81. **C) Health Insurance Portability and Accountability Act**

    The Health Insurance Portability and Accountability Act (HIPAA) was enacted in 1996. It is a federal law that requires the creation of national standards to protect sensitive patient health information from being disclosed without the patient's consent or knowledge. Healthcare organizations and professionals are required to exercise best practices in three areas: administrative, physical security, and technical security.

82. **A) Inability to perform complex problem-solving tasks**

    Noise and distractions can potentially increase the adverse effects on patient care outcomes, initiate poor task performance, and promote a decreased ability to concentrate, leading to an inability to perform complex problem-solving tasks. Healthcare personnel are usually able to perform simple problem-solving tasks until they start multi-tasking, especially when taking care of the patient. With noise and distractions, the nurse finds it more difficult to be able to perform simple and complex tasks related to direct patient care.

83. **C) Potassium 2.5 mEq/L**

    Low potassium levels prior to surgery have been associated with increased risk of adverse outcomes and perioperative mortality. A potassium value of 2.5 mEq/L is critically low and could present a risk for surgery. The surgery should be rescheduled until the patient's potassium value is raised to normal range. The hematocrit (HCT) value and platelet and white blood cell (WBC) counts are within normal range.

84. **C) Shelf life**

    Shelf life refers to the amount of time following the instrument sterilization process that a surgical item may be considered sterile. Proper handling, packaging, and storage can help to prevent contamination when standards and guidelines are followed.

85. **D) Immediate-type**

    An anaphylactic reaction is a type 1 hypersensitivity reaction, also known as an immediate-type allergic reaction. Allergies are divided into four different types: immediate-type, cytotoxic-type, immune complex-type, and delayed-type. Cytotoxic-type allergic reactions, type II, are mediated by IgG and IgM protein antibodies. They damage cells by the activation of the complement system, a component of the immune system. Immune complex-type allergic reactions, type III, are mediated by IgG and IgM protein antibodies and react along with the allergen to form antigen–antibody complexes, also known as immunocomplexes. These particular complexes are responsible for the reaction. Delayed-type allergic reactions, type IV, are also known as cell-mediated reactions. They are delayed because they usually occur 24 hours or longer after exposure to the allergen.

86. B) Ethical issues

The American Nurses Association (ANA) and the Association of periOperative Registered Nurses (AORN) have developed ethical guidelines that are considered nonnegotiable when caring for patients and families. These guidelines establish moral obligations to patients, the healthcare team, and the nursing profession as a whole. Legal, financial, and spiritual issues are not specifically addressed in the joint ANA and AORN guidelines.

87. A) First-intention healing

First-intention healing is the healing of a wound after primary closure that does not require further intervention. The skin is not damaged and the edges are well approximated to promote an optimal healing environment. Second-intention healing occurs when the wound heals by granulation, instead of being sutured closed. The wound heals spontaneously from the bottom up. Third-intention healing occurs when the suturing of the wound is delayed, the wound becomes infected, or the wound is too large to approximate the edges. Third-intention healing wounds need to be packed, and the patient requires antibiotic therapy to prevent/treat infection. Delayed primary closure is another name for third-intention healing.

88. C) Circulating nurse

The circulating nurse may work in all different phases of the perioperative setting—preoperative, intraoperative, and postoperative. The circulating nurse utilizes the nursing process in collaboration with the interdisciplinary team to coordinate the care of the patient through all phases of the surgical process. This is usually accomplished in areas where sterile surgical attire may not be necessary. The scrub nurse works within the boundaries of the operating room and assists in the care of the patient in the intraoperative environment. A float nurse is a nurse who can work in several different medical–surgical areas, depending on need. A float nurse is rarely used in the surgical setting. The advanced practice nurse refers to a nurse practitioner, nurse anesthetist, or clinical nurse specialist who is a member of the healthcare team and provides care to the patient in an advanced role, but does not coordinate the care in the perioperative setting.

89. C) Inner cap of pouring container

The inner cap of the pouring container is considered sterile, since it becomes exposed to the environment only when the container is opened. The outer cap is exposed to the environment; thus, it is not sterile. Spraying fluid is aerosolized, so it is not sterile due to exposure to the environment. The entire pouring container is not sterile since the outside of the container is exposed to the outside environment.

90. B) 6

The American Society of Anesthesiologists (ASA) physical (P) status classification scale includes six classifications for patients as it relates to their perioperative or peri-anesthesia risk and outcomes.

91. D) Repeat back important instructions

It is important to ensure that a patient understands their discharge instructions. The best method to evaluate if teaching has been successful is by asking the patient to repeat back important instructions. Asking the patient to sign a form and watch a video ensures that teaching has occurred, but does not validate that the patient understands. Asking the patient to verbally confirm that they understand the instructions is not sufficient.

92. D) Deliver a shock

Ventricular fibrillation (VF) is a shockable heart rhythm. According to the advanced cardiac life support (ACLS) pathway, the nurse would deliver a shock as soon as VF was noted on the heart monitor. This would be done regardless of the presence of a pulse. After the shock, the code team would resume CPR for 2 minutes, as well as evaluate and/or obtain intravenous/intraosseous infusion (IV/IO) access.

93. A) Patient safety

Situation, background, assessment, and recommendation (SBAR) is a hand-off tool that allows for collaborative and informative communication between nurses and other members of the multidisciplinary team. The main goal of hand-off communication is to provide continuity of care, which in turn promotes patient safety. SBAR is not used to promote confidentiality, infection control, and pain control.

94. A) Anxiety

A patient who asks questions repeatedly, withdraws from conversation, or avoids any communication is displaying characteristics of fear or anxiety, likely related to the impending surgical procedure. Depression or a knowledge deficit cannot conclusively be diagnosed at this time. The patient is not exhibiting characteristics of powerlessness.

95. C) The Association of periOperative Registered Nurses Accreditation Assistant

The Association of periOperative Registered Nurses (AORN) Accreditation Assistant is a comprehensive tool that was designed to help healthcare facilities be survey-ready by the time The Joint Commission (TJC) arrives to accredit the facility. It also provides a process to save staff preparation time. This tool maps each TJC standard/element of performance to the associated AORN guidelines, recommendations, and implementation tools. The AORN Accreditation Code, Accreditation Checklist, and Accreditation Guideline are all incorrect names for this survey-ready tool developed by AORN.

96. A) Ask the patient to describe the procedure in their own words

To evaluate how well the patient understands an upcoming procedure, the nurse should ask the patient to describe the procedure in their own words. The nurse can then provide feedback and clarify any misunderstandings. Witnessing a consent form does not evaluate a patient's comprehension of an upcoming procedure. Asking the patient questions about the surgery is not the most effective way to facilitate communication. Documenting that the patient received an educational brochure does not adequately evaluate a patient's comprehension of their upcoming surgery.

97. D) Perforations

Forceps have sharp, needle-like teeth that protrude from the ends to help grasp the skin. When forceps are grasped too tightly against the skin, they can create perforations, or buttonholes, in the skin. Scrapes are abrasions on the skin caused by friction. Burns require a source of heat. Bruising can be seen postop and signal bleeding underneath the skin.

98. A) A patient who received surgery on the wrong body part

A patient who received surgery on the wrong part of the body is an example of a sentinel event, which is an event that is unexpected and involves death or serious, permanent physical injury. Administering an extra dose of antibiotics to a patient is a medication error. The development of a wound infection should be investigated and follow-up actions implemented, but these are not considered sentinel events either.

99. **B) Scrub nurse**

    A scrub nurse functions as a member of the sterile team. The scrub nurse is responsible for maintaining a strict sterile atmosphere while handling surgical instruments and supplies. The scrub nurse works within the boundaries of the sterile OR and observes other members of the surgical team to ensure they maintain a sterile atmosphere. The circulating nurse is nonsterile and assists in positioning the patient on the OR bed, performing surgical scrubs with antimicrobial agents, assisting other members of the team with their duties, and counting instruments and sponges used during the surgical procedure. A first assistant nurse assists the surgeon during the procedure by exposing the surgical site and assisting with closure of the wound. The advanced practice nurse collaborates with members of the interdisciplinary team during all phases of the perioperative period and works to provide care management for the surgical patient.

100. **B) Environmental safety**

    Strategies promoting environmental safety include the recycling of certain perioperative waste and the proper disposal of hazardous, nonhazardous, and infectious materials. The maintenance of environmental safety through an effective perioperative waste management system also protects the healthcare workers, patients, and the community. This system could help to reduce financial costs, provided the policies and procedures are followed by the appropriate personnel.

101. **B) Document findings from the incident in the medical record using an objective manner.**

    The events of the situation should be documented in the patient's record, by the nurse, in an objective manner. The nurse should document the situation without adding bias and reasons that the family member might have acted the way that they did. The nurse should not speculate why the family member's demeanor suddenly changed. A nurse should document the facts without adding irrelevant information. Statements made by the patient and staff could be added and written in a subjective manner, but reactions should not be added due to the possibility of adding bias and personal reactions. The nurse should not record assumptions or conclusions regarding the family life of the patient; instead, the nurse should record only facts about the situation. An incident report could be mandated by the risk management department; however, the purpose of an incident report is not to reduce the incidence of malpractice suits filed by the family.

102. **B) 18 inches to 4 feet**

    The personal zone, which is 18 inches to 4 feet, is the optimal distance a nurse should sit from a patient during the interview phase. The intimate zone, which is 0 to 18 inches, is typically used with family and loved ones. The social zone, 4 to 12 feet, is used during interactions in the social or work atmosphere. The public zone, 12 to 25 feet, is used when speaking to small groups.

103. **D) Team education**

    According to the Association of periOperative Registered Nurses (AORN) position statement on environmental safety, best practices in regards to the environment can be developed and implemented in the perioperative area by educating the perioperative team, collaborating between the interdisciplinary team members, and by promoting advocacy. The best way for the nurse to encourage change to environmental practices is to educate the interdisciplinary team on why it is an important practice.

Education is important in the perioperative setting for patients and family members, but they are not involved in exposure to hazardous materials. They can educate them about recycling parameters in the surgical area. Physicians are members of the interdisciplinary team and would be a part of the team education in the best practices for environmental factors.

104. **C) The nurse is responsible for clarifying information about the procedure as required**
The nurse's role in the informed-consent process is to clarify information about the procedure as required. The surgeon is responsible for explaining the procedure and associated risks to the patient. The patient is responsible for signing the informed consent form, attesting that they understand all required information. The nurse may serve as a witness.

105. **B) Albumin**
Albumin levels indicate whether a patient is malnourished. Cholesterol, fasting glucose levels, and hemoglobin are not used to assess nutritional status.

106. **C) 12 hours**
The Association of periOperative Registered Nurses (AORN) recommends that a perioperative RN should not be required to work more than 12 consecutive hours in a 24-hour period. AORN also recommends that a perioperative nurse not work more than 60 hours in a 7-day work week. Working more than these two parameters can lead to increased emotional and physical stress and burnout and potentially compromise the safety of the nurse, patient, and interdisciplinary team members.

107. **A) Fatigue**
Human factors are those that affect the effectiveness of an individual's ability to safely perform the task at hand. In this scenario, a nurse who is fatigued may not be as alert or attentive during the surgery, and, in return, may not effectively communicate pertinent information as it relates to the procedure. The temperature of the room, background equipment noise, and intraoperative conversations are environmental factors.

108. **C) Asking the patient who is allowed to receive information about their care.**
All patient information should be held in confidentiality, according to the Health Insurance Portability and Accountability Act (HIPAA). The nurse should ask the patient who is allowed to receive information about their care. After establishing the patient's permission, the nurse can set up a passcode that would be required by the person(s) eliciting information. Providing information on a need-to-know basis and shredding any information no longer needed are acceptable actions, but not the best options in this scenario.

109. **C) Check the patient's chart for the documented vitals**
The most appropriate action by the nurse would be to check the patient's chart for the documented vitals. If the vitals are not documented (as they should be), the nurse should call the intraoperative nurse. The nurse should take the patient's vitals to create a baseline for postoperative care, but this should be done after the intraoperative vitals are obtained. It is never appropriate to ask a patient to provide their vitals.

110. **B) Introduction, patient, assessment, situation, safety concerns, the background, actions, timing, ownership, next**

    I PASS the BATON represents introduction, patient, assessment, situation, safety concerns, the background, actions, timing, ownership, and next. It is a mnemonic used for the promotion of effective patient hand-offs.

111. **B) High lithotomy**

    A radical perineal prostatectomy is a surgical procedure to completely remove the prostate from a small incision in the perineum, which is accessed with the patient's legs very high in stirrups with the knees near the ears (high lithotomy). Prone, low lithotomy, and lateral are not used in this type of surgery.

112. **C) Last menstrual cycle**

    It is important to ask the female patient about the date of her last menstrual cycle to rule out the possibility of pregnancy. Although questions may be asked about pregnancy history, birth control use, and most recent mammogram when relevant, the pregnancy status of ALL female patients must be determined prior to surgery.

113. **C) Place the Foley catheter preoperatively**

    A patient with a body mass index (BMI) of 41 has class 3 obesity, which may make placement of a Foley catheter more difficult and/or take more time than is usually required to place the catheter. The nurse should place the Foley catheter preoperatively to ensure there is ample time to place and address any complications that may arise. If the nurse waits to place the catheter in the OR, it may cut into valuable surgery time and cause delays for not only this surgery, but also other surgeries scheduled for the OR. While placement may be difficult, there are no factors that preclude the patient from receiving a Foley catheter; therefore, the nurse should not inform the surgeon that they cannot place the catheter. Nor should the nurse ask the surgeon to insert a suprapubic catheter, which is a surgical procedure completed under general anesthetic.

114. **C) Responsibility and accountability**

    Interdisciplinary team members in the surgical setting can most effectively deliver safe and effective care by being responsible and accountable. All members of the team must work together to ensure safe and efficient care of the patient, but each member is accountable for their own roles as a member of the team. Roles of each interdisciplinary team member should be established and clearly delineated. Any member of a team should display characteristics of reliability and sustainability, but they are not essential to delivering safe and effective care.

115. **C) Remove all instruments and restart with new sterile instruments**

    No instrument should be allowed to hang over the edge of the sterile field. If this occurs, the nurse should remove all instruments and restart with sterile instruments since it is now considered a contaminated environment. The nurse should not feel pressured about the surgery falling further behind schedule. Patient safety should always come first. Moving the forceps into the sterile field would further compromise the sterility. The sterile field should not be extended once instruments have already crossed over the edge. The nurse should not leave the forceps where they are. They are hanging over the sterile edge and are now considered contaminated.

116. **B) Circulating nurse and scrub nurse**

All healthcare personnel in the OR are responsible for making sure the surgical count is correct. However, the circulating nurse and the scrub nurse participate in several surgical counts together and each must initiate their own count to make sure both end up with the exact number of surgical items. This task must be done and documented to reduce the risk of an object being left inside a patient's body. A nurse anesthetist administers the anesthesia medications to the patient as ordered by an anesthesiologist. An advanced practice nurse may be in attendance but does not usually take on a role to initiate surgical counts. A physician is responsible for making sure the count is correct at the end of the procedure but does not initially start the count with the circulating nurse and scrub nurse.

117. **D) Vibrio**

A type-III necrotizing fasciitis is caused by waterborne microorganisms, which are vibrio. Type-I necrotizing fasciitis are aerobic and anaerobic. Beta-hemolytic streptococcus is an example of type-II necrotizing fasciitis, the most common type.

118. **B) When the glove is pulled over the sleeve**

All of these scenarios could promote contamination and cross-contamination, but the most concerning is when gloves are pulled over the gown. This can cause a nurse to have false security that fluids are less likely to leak through the PPE and may result in less vigilance. When the glove rolls down or slips on the sleeve, the risk of exposure to blood or body fluids increases, but the nurse is more likely to identify that the glove has slipped or rolled and fix the issue. Although there are some personal protective equipment (PPE) with anti-slip properties offered in the marketplace, the interface between the gown and the glove remains vulnerable to fluid leaks.

119. **C) Chemicals of concern**

Chemicals of concern are described in the Association of periOperative Registered Nurses (AORN) position statement on environmental responsibility. Chemicals of concern are designated by the United States Environmental Protection Agency (EPA) as chemicals that are persistent, toxic, bioaccumulative, and known to be carcinogenic or suspected to be carcinogenic. Air toxins can be noncarcinogenic substances, as well as carcinogenic substances. Waste products are not necessarily chemicals and are not listed by the EPA. The waste stream refers to the flow of discarded fluids.

120. **D) A woman who takes daily anticoagulants to treat atrial fibrillation**

All of these medications and situations would be assessed and reviewed at some level. The medication regimen that has the highest priority would be the woman who takes daily anticoagulants to treat atrial fibrillation. She would need to be assessed for bleeding and have labs drawn (including prothrombin time/international normalized ratio [PT/INR]) that would need to be evaluated as soon as possible. If the INR level was higher than the surgeon is comfortable with, the surgery may need to be canceled due to an increased risk for excessive bleeding. A patient who takes nonsteroidal anti-inflammatory drugs (NSAIDs) would need to be asked which specific NSAID is used and the number of tablets/capsules taken daily. The woman taking the thyroid medication and the man taking the ACE inhibitor would be assessed, but they would not require a more specific preoperative assessment than the woman on anticoagulants.

121. **D) 825 mL/hr**

According to the American Society of Regional Anesthesia and Pain Medicine (ASRA) protocol for lipid emulsion 20%, the infusion rate for a patient who weighs less than 70 kg is 0.25 mL/kg/min. The patient in this scenario weighs 55 kg; thus, the rate would be 825 mL/hr.

122. **C) Preprocedural checklist**

During the preoperative stage, the use of preprocedural checklists helps to prevent emergency situations by ensuring that important patient characteristics, including allergies and previous anesthesia reactions, are not overlooked. The time-out and briefing period is a part of the comprehensive surgical checklist, which is used to improve communication among the surgical team. They take place in the intraoperative period.

123. **C) Ignition source**

The three components of an OR fire are oxidizers, ignition sources, and fuel sources. Oxidizers are solids, liquids, or gases that can intensify combustion and increase the flammable range for chemicals so they ignite more readily. Examples of oxidizers include oxygen and nitrous oxide. Ignition sources include medical equipment such as lasers, drills, electrosurgical devices, and scopes. Fuel sources include combustible materials such as alcohol-containing liquids, sponges and gauze, drapes, endotracheal tubes, and nasal cannula.

124. **A) History of varicosities**

Risks for development of a deep vein thrombus include a personal or family history of thrombosis, coagulopathy, blood clots, blood clotting disorders, previous deep vein thrombosis, pulmonary embolism, varicosities, smoking, or sedentary lifestyle. Alcohol abuse, upper respiratory infection, and increased body mass index do not increase the risk of deep vein thrombosis.

125. **D) Feelings of intimidation**

The OR culture is often not conducive to effective communication because team members may feel intimidated about speaking up, even when they are aware of problems that need to be addressed. Lack of knowledge, credibility, and limited skill sets may lead to an error; however, they are not a result of an OR culture.

126. **D) Anxiety, fear, knowledge**

The nurse working in the preoperative setting should set a tone and provide activities to decrease anxiety, decrease fear, and increase knowledge. These three areas have been shown to assist in decreasing complications following a surgical procedure. It also promotes physical and psychologic healing following surgery. The nurse can assist the patient with utilizing optimistic and positive statements to help with decreasing the levels of pain, anxiety, and fear. The nurse will conduct an assessment and obtain medical history, including nutritional status, allergies, family history, and pain level. This information is important to obtain and the surgery should not commence until these assessments are completed. However, the nurse should assist the patient in decreasing anxiety and fear and increasing their knowledge in how to promote a healthy postoperative environment.

127. **C) Less than 1 mcg/kg**

     The recommended dosage for epinephrine in resuscitation of patients with local anesthetic systemic toxicity (LAST) is less than 1 mcg/kg. Dosage of 1,000 mcg or 1 mg is the recommended dosage for resuscitation of a patient without LAST as a part of the advanced cardiac life support (ACLS) protocol. Dosages of 5,000 mcg and greater than 1 mcg/kg are not recommendations of either protocol.

128. **A) To help the patient return to their baseline**

     The peri-anesthesia nurse's role is to help the patient return to a safe physiologic state after receiving any form of anesthesia. Assisting the patient with discharge and self-care is performed by the pre- and postoperative staff. Peri-anesthesia nurses do assess for complications postoperatively.

129. **A) Sterilization**

     Spaulding's classification scheme has several categories that work together to determine the correct processing methods for surgical items and devices. According to this scheme, if the item comes into contact with any sterile tissue or the vascular system, it is considered to be a critical item and should be sterilized. Examples of these items include needles, surgical instruments, catheters, and cutting endoscopic accessories. Items that come into contact with nonintact skin or mucous membranes are considered semi-critical items and should be sterilized or undergo a minimum of high-level disinfection. Examples of these types of items are respiratory therapy equipment, gastrointestinal scopes, and bronchoscopes. Items that are considered to be noncritical items are those that come into contact with intact skin. These items require intermediate-level disinfection, low-level disinfection, or cleaning. Examples of these items include nondisposable blood pressure cuffs, linens, and surgical suite furnishings.

130. **B) Vital signs**

     The "S" in SBAR stands for situation, which includes vital signs. The "B" stands for background, which includes information about the patient's mental status, skin condition, and oxygen status. The "A" stands for assessment, which includes current physical findings. The "R" stands for recommendations, which include physician recommendations and required tests.

131. **A) The patient's educational level**

     When developing an educational program or plan for a postoperative patient, it is most important to consider the patient's educational level, which would include literacy. The nurse needs to be aware of how the information should be communicated to facilitate learning. Although it is important to assess the patient's relationship with their spouse to determine if reinforcement can be done by the spouse, it is not the most important. While it is important to inquire about additional support after discharge in the event the patient has additional needs beyond the spouse's capability, it is not most important in the stage of developing their initial educational plan. Their schedule is not relevant to the development of the plan.

132. **B) The anesthesia is not adequate, and the dose needs to be adjusted.**

     Anesthesia should keep the patient comfortable, sedated, and paralyzed, with minimal fluctuation in vital signs. It is not normal for the patient to move during surgery or to have a sudden increase in the heart rate. Therefore, the patient may not be sedated enough, and the dose needs to be adjusted. The patient is not having an adverse reaction; instead, the anesthesia is wearing off. They should receive more medication and continue the surgery with caution. This is not a normal phenomenon that occurs during induction of anesthesia.

133. **C) Reverse cut**

A reverse-cut needle is preferred for subcutaneous suturing. When it transects the skin lateral to the wall on the outside, the cutting edge points away from the wound edge, and the inside flat edge is parallel to the edge of the wound, thereby reducing the tendency for the suture to tear through tissue. Blunt, Keith, and taper-cut sutures are not preferred for subcutaneous suturing.

134. **A) Maintaining airway**

The nurse's first priority in trauma patients is maintaining airway. Priority management in trauma patients is as follows: Establish and maintain airway and ventilation, control hemorrhage, prevent and treat hypovolemic shock, assess for head and neck injuries, and complete other assessments and diagnostics. Therefore, minimizing pain and blood loss, starting an intravenous line (IV), initiating any fluids, and drawing and type screen and match would only occur after maintaining a patent airway.

135. **B) Move the arm away from the body to allow access to the left side intercostal spaces**

A left lateral thoracotomy involves incising the left intercostal spaces to reach the heart for repair. The left arm is abducted and moved away from the body laterally to promote access to the left side intercostal spaces. Moving the arm closer to the body would be adduction. The arm is not moved anteriorly, in front of the body, as this would occlude the surgeon's field. The angle of 70 degrees is safe and effectively prevents brachial nerve plexus injury. If the arm is abducted more than 90 degrees, which is hyperabduction, it may injure the brachial nerve.

136. **A) Fear**

Fear is the most common psychosocial emotion displayed during the preoperative phase. This fear is usually associated with the unknown and perceived lack of control. It is not common for the preoperative patient to have anger, depression, or frustration. These are sometimes seen postoperatively related to the surgical procedure performed and patient's ability to recover.

137. **B) Apply a cloth barrier to the arm under the blood pressure cuff**

A cloth barrier can be placed on the patient's arm, under the blood pressure (BP) cuff, when taking BP. This prevents the skin from coming into contact with the cuff in the case of an allergic reaction. Tubing made with polyvinyl chloride is safe to use with a latex allergy and is the tubing of choice in this situation. Medications from glass ampules are safe to use in patients with a latex allergy. Medications from ampules with rubber stoppers are contraindicated in patients with a latex allergy. The nurse should also follow the policy and procedure of the medical facility for a patient with a latex allergy.

138. **A) Hulka tenaculum**

The Hulka tenaculum is an instrument that raises the uterus and clamps onto the cervix to open the canal and allow contrast media to be instilled. Vise-grip pliers are used to stabilize bone during orthopedic surgeries. Curettes and gouges are debulking instruments used to remove tissue.

139. **C) "What do you think you should do?"**

The nurse should use the techniques of reflection to allow the patient to explore their feelings about having the amputation. The nurse should not suggest how the patient should proceed as this would be giving advice, which should be avoided. The nurse would be giving approval by stating "I think you should have it." This is discouraged as it may influence the patient's decision. Suggesting that all patients "feel this way" before amputation surgery is dismissive and belittling to the patient.

140. **B) Epinephrine**

Epinephrine is the first line of treatment for acute anaphylaxis, followed by the administration of corticosteroids and H1 (e.g., hydroxyzine) and H2 antihistamines. Epinephrine works to relax the muscles that are blocking the airways by binding to the receptors on smooth muscles. This allows the breathing of the patient to return to normal. Dantrolene is the antidote drug for malignant hyperthermia and is not a drug used to treat anaphylaxis.

141. **B) Montgomery strap**

Montgomery straps are adhesive bandages that have gauze string attached to one end to secure bulky dressings in place. Stockinette is tubed knitted cotton that is placed over extremities before applying gauze. Nonallergenic tape is used to secure dressings in place. Four-ply crinkle gauze is a type of elastic bandage.

142. **C) "ICS maximizes inflation of your lungs and reduces the risk of pneumonia."**

An incentive spirometer maximizes the inflation of the patient's lungs and reduces/prevents atelectasis, which can lead to pneumonia. It is a way for patients to promote deep breathing following surgery and gives a visual feedback so the patient can determine how they are progressing with their deep-breathing exercises. The goal for the patient is to gradually increase the amount of air inhaled. ICS does not completely diminish the risk of pneumonia but it does reduce or decrease the incidence for pneumonia.

143. **B) Cycle outlined in manufacturer's instructions for the set and container**

Cleaning and handling instructions can vary depending on the device manufacturer. Some instruments, especially powered instruments, require special cleaning and maintenance procedures. The appropriate cycle for immediate-use steam sterilization (IUSS) would be determined after review of the manufacturer's recommendations. OSHA standards do not specifically address IUSS.

144. **C) 6 to 12 months**

According to the Association of periOperative Registered Nurses (AORN) position statement on orientation of the registered nurses and surgical technologists in the perioperative setting, the length of a complete orientation of the surgical setting is 6 to 12 months. The orientation should include didactic learning and a clinical component. While a generalized orientation program can serve as a base study, each orientation should be individualized depending on the job functions and duties of the novice nurse.

145. **D) Autologous**

A patient who donates their own blood in the event they require an intraoperative or postoperative blood transfusion is giving an *autologous donation*. When the patient's family and friends donate blood for their exclusive use, it is a *direct blood donation. Homologous* and *heterologous* refer to blood transfusions, not blood donations. Homologous is the collection and infusion of blood from a compatible donor and heterologous transfusions are those that involve infusing blood from a different species.

146. **C) Before the patient enters the surgical suite**
The position statement by the Association of periOperative Registered Nurses (AORN) notes that prevention for pressure injuries should occur before the patient enters the surgical suite. The preoperative nurse should conduct a risk factor assessment and obtain a medical history and physical assessment to determine risk factors that might predispose the patient to a higher risk of pressure injuries during surgery. The perioperative staff should have annual education and training regarding pressure injury prevention in the surgical setting. Waiting until the patient is in surgery and directly after surgery is too late to assess the patient's risk for pressure injury and too late to start interventions for prevention. Twenty-four hours after surgery is also too late to start the prevention of pressure injuries that can occur during surgery. Preventing pressure injuries should be a priority for the interdisciplinary team, and the assessment findings should be communicated to all members of the healthcare team at every handoff session.

147. **B) "The glasses you are wearing are not sufficient."**
During any surgery requiring the use of a laser, the staff's and patient's eyes must be protected with glasses that wrap around the side of their face or goggles that prevent damage from the laser. Regular eyeglasses do not offer sufficient protection because they do not cover the top, bottom, and sides of the visual field. Eyeglass tinting does not offer any protection. The protective eye goggles would be sterilized.

148. **C) Association for the Advancement of Medical Instrumentation**
The Association for Advancement of Medical Instrumentation (AAMI) offers standards, guidelines, and recommendations for central processing and sterilization of medical and surgical instruments. The American Society of PeriAnesthesia Nurses, ASPAN, has issued standards and guidelines specific to the area of perianesthesia that provide a framework for the scope of care for these patients. It includes position statements and recommendations for practice in perianesthesia. IAHCSMM is the International Association of Healthcare Central Service Material Management. APIC is the Association for Professionals in Infection Control and Epidemiology.

149. **A) Hypercarbia**
Malignant hyperthermia (MH) is a type of severe reaction that occurs in response to use of general anesthetics. It occurs in patients who are susceptible to the condition due to a number of factors (e.g., inherited muscle diseases). Hypercarbia is the earliest and most sensitive sign of MH. Muscle rigidity is the most specific. The other initial symptoms, such as tachycardia and tachypnea, are nonspecific and thus not the most sensitive signs for diagnosing MH.

150. **D) Assess the patient for any physiologic changes and alert the surgical team**
Sudden change in mentation and refusing the surgery is a red flag. The nurse should assess the patient for any physiologic changes and alert the surgical team that the patient has changed their mind. The nurse should not tell the patient it is too late to cancel. If the patient is refusing the surgery, the nurse cannot forcibly bring the patient to the OR. Administering a medication to sedate the patient and make them more agreeable is unethical.

151. **A) As soon as possible**
According to the Association of periOperative Registered Nurses (AORN) Explication for the American Nurses Association (ANA) Code of Ethics, the perioperative nurse should act as an advocate for the patient when they are determining the specific healthcare decisions they want to follow. This promotes their independence, dignity, and rights as a human. However, when it becomes necessary to override the wishes of the patient to save their life or follow regulatory requirements, the patient's rights are suspended until they can be restored—as soon as possible. This restoration does not require an order from the physician.

152. **D) At the point of use during the surgical procedure**
According to the AORN guidelines, decontamination of surgical instruments should begin at the point of use (POU) during the surgery. This helps to prevent or decrease the amount of dried material on the instruments. In turn, this should improve the cleaning process by increasing the efficacy and effectiveness of the overall cleaning procedure.

153. **D) Pre-procedure**
It is during the pre-procedure process that the perioperative nurse asks the patient about any special equipment or implants.

154. **C) Metallic taste**
According to the classic progression of clinical signs and symptoms of local anesthetic systemic toxicity (LAST), metallic taste would be among the initial symptoms. Latter symptoms include confusion, respiratory depression, and then hypertension.

155. **C) Ethylene oxide gas**
Ethylene oxide gas (ETO) is a chemical agent that interferes with cell metabolism and reproduction of the cell. Although it is a flammable chemical and explosive, it does not require high heat and leaves no residue on the instruments. Ozone gas damages cell membranes, which leads to destruction of the cells. Hydrogen peroxide vapor damages cell membranes as well as cell systems involving enzyme activity. Peracetic acid destroys cell proteins, which leads to death of the cell.

156. **C) Has friable skin**
Friable skin/tissue is fragile and bleeds easily. The removal of tape and subsequent bleeding is a sign that a patient has friable skin. A hypertrophic scar is raised from the skin. Occlusive dressings allow air passage but not fluids. This patient would not require an occlusive dressing simply because of their friable skin. Wound dehiscence is a splitting and reopening of a wound.

157. **D) Tell the anesthesiologist that administration poses a safety risk**
Telling the anesthesiologist that administration poses a safety risk is practicing assertive communication, which should be used when challenges arise during the intraoperative phases. Telling the anesthesiologist they are wrong and questioning their choice can be perceived as undermining and challenging their knowledge. This would create a barrier to communication. Telling the anesthesiologist they are going to kill the patient is aggressive communication, which should never be used in a professional setting.

158. B) One

The position statement of the Association of periOperative Registered Nurses (AORN) regarding safe staffing states that a minimum of one perioperative RN circulator should be assigned to every patient scheduled for a surgical and/or invasive procedure.

159. C) Nonverbal

Nonverbal communication often relies on facial expressions and hand and body gestures, which are not conducive to the OR environment and may lead to miscommunication and an increase in stress levels. Intraoperative team members are required to wear masks that cover most of their faces, limiting recognition of facial expressions. In addition, intraoperative team members are often multitasking, which can make it difficult to see or understand hand or body gestures. The most effective communication in the OR is closed-loop communication, which requires a call-out and check-back method to confirm that messages and orders are correct and understood. Formal and written communication would not cause miscommunication in the OR as they provide a clear and consistent form of communication between team members.

160. C) Beta blockers

Abrupt discontinuation of a beta blocker could result in a dangerous increase in blood pressure, which could lead to fatal outcomes; therefore, beta-blocker use should continue up to and sometimes even during surgery. It is important to document the time the last dose was taken in the event it needs to be taken before surgery. It is not necessary to document the time of last dose for anti-arrhythmias, angiotensin-converting enzyme (ACE) inhibitors, and loop diuretics.

161. B) Relative humidity can impact the shelf life and product integrity of sterile supplies.

Relative humidity (RH) can impact the shelf life and product integrity of sterile supplies in the OR. The American Society of Heating, Refrigeration, and Air Conditioning Engineers (ASHRAE) sets the international standard for heating, ventilation, and air conditioning (HVAC) parameters for RH, which state that the RH for surgical and procedure settings with anesthesia should be between 20% to 60%. These parameters are supported by the American Society for Healthcare Engineering (ASHE), the Association of periOperative Registered Nurses (AORN), and The Joint Commission (TJC). RH has not been researched on nonsterile supplies since all of the supplies used in the OR are sterile.

162. B) Hemostat

Occluding instruments are used to stop bleeding, or cut off/occlude blood flow. Hemostat is an occluding instrument. Scalpel and scissors are dissecting instruments. Forceps are grasping instruments.

163. B) Marking the site for surgery

Marking the site for surgery is an element of surgical "time-out," which is a final reassurance of accurate patient identity, surgical site, and planned procedure. This process promotes patient safety and reduces the risk of error and adverse events. Preparing a sterile field and ensuring that lighting is adequate for surgery is promotion of a healthy environment and does not reduce the risk of adverse effects. Reviewing the preadmission checklist is a task completed by the surgical team before a procedure, not the surgeon. Information may be documented incorrectly and may lead to an adverse event if not clarified and validated.

164. B) Potassium

An abnormal potassium level (less than 3.5 mEq/L) could cause cardiac arrhythmia during surgery. Abnormal sodium, hemoglobin, and fasting blood glucose levels can cause intraoperative complications, but they are not usually associated with arrhythmias.

165. C) Tell the anesthesiologist

There are multiple factors that need to be considered when selecting appropriate anesthesia drugs and amount used. The anesthesiologist should be made aware of the patient's heavy use of valium as this will impact the amount required to induce anesthesia and keep the patient comfortably sedated during surgery. The lead surgeon can be made aware of the patient's anxiety and use of valium, but the anesthesiologist controls the sedation during the procedure and should be the priority individual to inform. The nurse can make a note in the patient's chart, but it is a higher priority to inform the anesthesiologist. While it is appropriate to speak to the patient about their anxiety, the nurse should not provide false assurances.

166. A) Chemical indicator

The Bowie-Dick test, or daily air-removal test (DART), is a chemical indicator that is reviewed every day before the first load of instruments is processed for sterilization. This test demonstrates that air is being eliminated from the chamber of each air-removal autoclave. Physical monitors include gauges that record activities in the chamber, recordings of temperature and pressure, and digital printouts. A biologic monitor determines if microorganisms have been destroyed and is the most accurate method for proving proper sterilization has been achieved. There is no sterilization monitor system that is called a pressure indicator.

167. B) Lumbar spine

The Association of periOperative Registered Nurses (AORN) has created and implemented guidelines on safety to protect the patient and the healthcare worker. These guidelines recommend that the operating room (OR) environment develop a systemized program.

168. A) Horizontal violence

According to the Association of periOperative Registered Nurses (AORN) and the position statement on a healthy perioperative practice environment, horizontal violence is chronic behavior that occurs between coworkers on an organizational level that is disruptive, unkind, and disrespectful. Horizontal violence is also called lateral violence. It includes gossip, sabotage, and sarcasm. The definition of incivility is behavior that is disrespectful, rude, and inconsiderate. The definition of bullying involves persistent and repeated verbal, nonverbal, and physical acts. Horizontal violence can become abuse when the behaviors escalate to verbal and physical acts.

169. B) Continue to take as directed

Phenobarbital use should be maintained to prevent seizure activity during surgery. Discontinuing the use of an antiseizure medication before surgery would increase the risk of seizure activity during surgery.

170. A) Plume

While lasers do have benefits, there are risk factors associated with their use, including fire and damage to the eyes, as well as biologic hazards to the eyes such as laser plume. Lasers are utilized to decrease surgical site infections and reduce blood loss in the postoperative patient. Mechanical failure, electrical shortage, and electrical shock could all be possibilities when working with lasers but they would not be considered biologic hazards to laser utilization. The surgical department would need to have at least one perioperative nurse complete training as a laser safety officer (LSO) and certification as a certified LSO (CLSO). This person would be responsible for administering the laser safely.

171. D) Destroy organisms before they enter the body.

Surgical asepsis refers to the destruction of bacteria, or microbes, before they enter the body. Surgical asepsis does not occur when bacteria, or microbes, leave the body. Isolating any patient that has an infectious disease and maintaining all areas for basic cleanliness both refer to medical asepsis, not surgical asepsis.

172. D) Diagnostic

Diagnostic is a term used to classify a surgical procedure that determines the origin and cause of a disorder. Radical is an example of a term used to describe the extent of a surgery. Emergent is an example of a term used to describe the urgency of a surgery, and minor is an example of a term used to describe the degree of risk the surgery poses to the patient.

173. B) Mentoring

The experienced nurse is mentoring the novice nurse by providing regular support, guidance, and advice via monthly meetings. Mentoring is a vital process in nursing as it facilitates the acclimation of novice nurses to their new role and helps them develop their skills. Formal mentorship relationships in nursing typically take place over a 6- to 12-month period. While managers often play the role of mentor, the manager–employee relationship is ongoing and includes other elements such as performance assessment and evaluation. Advocacy refers to an action that speaks in favor of, recommends, supports, or defends an individual or a specific cause or organization. A preceptorship is typically a short-term assignment that provides orientation to a particular unit, with a focus on the development and evaluation of clinical skills. Nursing students are precepted in the clinical setting to ensure clinical competence before graduation.

174. B) Surgical procedure, wet, instruments, tissue, counts, have you any questions

SWITCH stands for surgical procedure, wet (e.g., fluids), instruments, tissue (e.g., specimen), counts, have you any questions. It is a tool used to convey important information in hand-offs.

175. A) Herbal

Herbal medications are often not considered medications to patients; therefore, they fail to report them. The nurse should specifically ask the patient about the use of these medications. Prescribed medications, such as psychiatric and cardiovascular medications, are often reported by the patient during the medication use assessment.

176. **C) 3 minutes**

The minimum recommended drying time for alcohol-based preps is 3 minutes, which helps to reduce the incidence of operating room fires.

177. **C) Interpersonal communication**

Interpersonal communication involves two or more people who work together to exchange information. In the perioperative environment, it can include the nurse, patient, family members, and participants in the interdisciplinary team. Intrapersonal communication is referred to as *self-talk* and involves communication within a single person. Organizational communication occurs when a group of people within a certain organization communicate together to work toward a common goal. Group communication is communication within a small group.

178. **C) They improve patient outcomes**

Supply management issues can greatly impact the efficiency of the perioperative area and patient safety. An efficient inventory management system ultimately serves to improve patient outcomes (including patient safety) and decrease costs. An inventory management system is used to manage supply issues; it is not used for sterilization, staffing, or for environmental purposes.

179. **B) Malignant hyperthermia**

King-Denborough syndrome is a genetic condition and is a form of congenital myopathy. Patients with a personal or family history of this condition may be at increased risk for malignant hyperthermia. This condition does not put the patient at increased risk for an anaphylactic reaction, hypothermia, or hypoxemia.

180. **B) Local anesthetic systemic toxicity**

The acronym LAST stands for local anesthetic systemic toxicity. LAST is a life-threatening adverse event that may occur after the administration of local anesthetic drugs through a variety of routes. Initial signs and symptoms include agitation, confusion, dizziness, drowsiness, dysphoria, auditory changes, tinnitus, perioral numbness, metallic taste, and dysarthria.

181. **D) Advance directive**

It is essential for the healthcare staff to know the status of a patient's advance directive before surgery. The advance directive is a legal document that explains the patient's wishes for care, as well as appoints a person to make decisions if the patient should become unable to do so. If something were to happen during the surgical process, the advance directive would indicate the patient's wishes, but in most cases, the physician must translate that directive into an actual hospital order, such as a DNR order, if indicated and the physician felt that was appropriate. Prior to surgery, the patient should notify the physician that he has an advance directive, as well as give a copy of the advance directive to the admitting nurse. The patient should have a copy of the advance directive, and if there is a designated power of attorney for medical decisions that should be noted as well. Copies of these documents should be placed on the chart and become a part of the permanent record. Power of attorney designates the person(s) to make decisions about property, finances, or medical care. A general will is a document that directs how a person wants their assets distributed following their death. A healthcare proxy is a legal document that designates someone to make all of the medical decisions for them in an urgent or emergency situation. The patient would be unable to state their medical wishes in those specific situations and it would be conducted by a healthcare proxy.

182. **D) Wedge under right hip**

A wedge should be placed under the right hip as it displaces the uterus off the inferior vena cava, protecting the fetal blood supply. Lateral, wedge under left hip, and supine are not appropriate due to potential for diminished blood supply to the fetus.

183. **C) Extent and role of the patient's support network**

The nurse needs to obtain a psychosocial assessment during the initial history assessment and this can include spiritual and cultural information as well. Psychosocial distress occurs in many different forms with patients. Some patients ask a lot of questions, and some patients may be quiet and reserved. Some patients may appear very anxious, while other patients may appear more depressed. Patients who have a focused and supportive network of family members, friends, church members, and/or spiritual advisors tend to have more positive outcomes than patients who do not have this type of supportive network. The healthcare provider, community resources, and insurance carrier are important, but they do not provide more positive outcomes for the patient than a supportive network.

184. **D) American Society of Regional Anesthesia and Pain Medicine**

The acronym ASRA stands for the American Society of Regional Anesthesia and Pain Medicine, which provides guidelines and advisories for complication of regional anesthesia.

185. **C) Sterile items should be stored in covered carts or closed cabinets when outside a sterile room.**

The Association of periOperative Registered Nurses (AORN) Guidelines for Sterilization recommend that sterile items must be stored in closed cabinets or carts that are covered when outside a sterile room. This helps to reduce the risk of sterile item contamination. The recommendation does not specify that sterile items should be locked or double locked. Sterile equipment and medical devices must have an expiration date; otherwise, they would be considered non-sterile.

186. **B) Occlude the esophagus to allow stabilization**

Compressing the cricoid cartilage, also known as Sellick's maneuver, is used to occlude the esophagus and promote stabilization of the trachea to assist with intubation. The airway is not occluded when doing this maneuver. The trachea should not move when the patient is sedated; it is not necessary to hold it in place. The anesthesiologist locates the trachea by placing the scope into the throat and visualizing it.

187. **D) Composition of aspirate and volume of the aspirate**

One of the risks during surgery with general anesthesia is aspiration, which can occur when liquid and/or solid material is regurgitated from the stomach and enters the lung. Different pulmonary syndromes can occur following aspiration with associated hypoxia, acute respiratory distress syndrome (ARDS), respiratory failure, and death. Composition of the aspirate and the volume of the aspirate are contributing factors. Aspiration during anesthesia occurs due to insufficient reflexes of the larynx that would normally protect the airway from regurgitation of liquids and/or solid material. The pulmonary syndromes that can occur are ARDS, pneumonitis, airway obstruction, pneumonia, and cardiopulmonary collapse leading to death. The length of time since the patient's last meal could increase the risk but it would not assist in determining what pulmonary syndrome developed from the aspiration. A history of gastric ulcer and history of acid-reflux disease in the patient would be important components of the medical history of the patient, but neither would help to determine what pulmonary syndrome will result from the actual aspiration.

188. C) Maintain aseptic conditions and process equipment

The primary responsibility of a scrub nurse is to maintain aseptic conditions for the patient and surgical team while in the OR. This includes making certain that all equipment that will be utilized is sterile and that all OR personnel maintain a sterile environment. The scrub nurse also processes all equipment. The scrub nurse works within the surgical suite and does not rotate between the holding area during preoperative activities and does not maintain the patient in the postoperative area. The preoperative nurse would be responsible for educating the patient regarding discharge medications and measures to prevent possible postoperative complications. The preoperative nurse or an advanced practice nurse would be responsible for completing the health assessment and formulating the initial nursing care plan.

189. B) Dantrolene

Malignant hyperthermia (MH) is a type of severe reaction that occurs in response to use of general anesthetics. It occurs in patients who are susceptible to the condition due to a number of factors (e.g., inherited muscle diseases). Dantrolene is a muscle relaxer that is used to treat MH. Tizanidine, metaxalone, and methocarbamol are muscle relaxers as well, but they are not used to treat MH.

190. A) Silence

Silence is a communication technique used to give the patient the opportunity to collect and organize their thoughts, as well as think through a point. Acceptance conveys reception and regard to what is being said by the patient. Focusing is taking one point of a conversation and highlighting it to explore further, and reflecting involves questions referred back to the patient to validate their point of view.

191. D) Speaking in clichés

A cliché is a common, trite statement that gives the impression that the nurse is not taking the patient's concerns seriously. Clichés should be avoided in therapeutic communication. Other ways to impede therapeutic communication with a patient are changing the subject and being judgmental. Giving advice, even when the patient asks, should be avoided as well as it is inappropriate for a nurse to provide a patient with advice.

192. A) Hydrogen

Hydrogen, a gastrointestinal gas, is a patient-dependent fuel source in OR fires. Other patient-dependent fuel sources include hair and soft tissue. Acetone, benzoin, and ether are patient-independent fuel sources.

193. B) Regional anesthesia

Regional anesthesia is directed at the nerves in the surgical area. This allows the patient to remain awake and aware of their surroundings during the procedure. Patients may be given medications with regional anesthesia for mild sedation and/or to decrease anxiety. General anesthesia renders a patient asleep, unarousable, and unaware of their surroundings. With local anesthesia, a solution is injected directly into the tissues surrounding the injection site. Intravenous anesthesia is used to induce and maintain general anesthesia.

194. A) Correct site? Correct equipment?

The surgical time-out includes a list of questions to prevent the wrong site of surgery. Questions address correct site and correct equipment. Correct location (or OR) and correct staff are not included on the list. The list also includes correct images and correct procedure.

195. A) Patient with severe liver disease

Patients with severe liver disease are most vulnerable to local anesthetic systemic toxicity (LAST) with amide local anesthetics such as lidocaine. Patients with respiratory acidosis, ischemic heart disease, and end-stage renal disease may develop LAST, but not specific to amide local anesthetics.

196. C) Hypotension and bronchospasm

Anaphylaxis often presents with bronchospasm and/or hypotension. For this reason, it is often misdiagnosed because many disorders may present with these same symptoms. Hypertension, tachycardia, and bradycardia are not typical symptoms of anaphylaxis.

197. C) The Joint Commission

The Joint Commission (TJC) is responsible for accrediting and certifying healthcare facilities in the United States. The Association of periOperative Nurses (AORN) developed a comprehensive tool, the Accreditation Assistant, to help healthcare facilities be ""survey-ready"" for TJC site visit. This tool addresses each TJC standard and elements of performance and has versions for each TJC program including Ambulatory, Critical Access Hospital, Hospital and Office-Based Surgery, and the Sterile Processing Department. The Centers for Medicare and Medicaid Services (CMS) is a federal agency that administers the Medicare, Medicaid, and CHIP programs. The Occupational Safety and Health Administration (OSHA) provides standards for how to prevent exposure to contaminated blood products and hazardous chemicals in the intraoperative area. The Centers for Disease Control and Prevention (CDC) develops and applies disease prevention and control, environmental health, and health promotion and health education activities.

198. C) Phase III

According to the established standards of American Society of PeriAnesthesia Nurses (ASPAN), patients in phase III are ready for discharge. The pre-anesthesia phase occurs before surgery. The postanesthesia phase I focuses on immediate postoperative care such as in the recovery room. Postanesthesia phase II focuses on extended care of the patient, such as transferring to a unit within the hospital. There are only three phases of established standards.

199. A) Attending to the patient's needs and performing a review of body systems

The circulating nurse is responsible for the patient once the patient is brought into the OR, including attending to the patient's needs and performing a brief review of systems (ROS). The surgeon is responsible for marking the surgical site with their initials. The scrub person should continue to prepare the OR while the circulating nurse tends to the patient. The entire team's attention should not be directed to the patient until the ROS is complete and they have finished prepping supplies and scrubbing in.

200. **D) Abdominal aortic aneurysm repair**

Abdominal aortic aneurysm (AAA) has the highest rate of postoperative respiratory failure when compared to other surgeries, including thoracic procedures. A craniotomy or cholecystectomy has not been associated with postoperative respiratory failure. Femoral-popliteal bypass surgery is associated with higher cardiac adverse reactions.

12 ANSWERS TO POP QUIZZES AND UNFOLDING SCENARIOS

CHAPTER 2

UNFOLDING SCENARIO 2.1A

Assessment of the documentation associated with the surgery is required (e.g., history and physical, laboratory and diagnostic results, informed consent, and anesthesia consent).

POP QUIZ 2.1

The anesthesiologist should be made aware that the surgical site is not marked, and the nerve block will need to be delayed. The surgeon will need to be contacted and asked to mark the patient.

UNFOLDING SCENARIO 2.1B

Alert the team that the time-out has not been performed. Ask all members of the team to pause so that this important action can be completed.

UNFOLDING SCENARIO 2.1C

Alert the team that the patient has not been securely strapped. Ask the scrub technician to carefully move away. Place the strap across the thighs. The belt must be out of the way of the surgical field.

POP QUIZ 2.2

The circulating nurse should alert the anesthesiologist and the surgeon right away. The surgical site marking should be consistent with the patient's confirmation of the procedure and the contents of the surgical consent.

POP QUIZ 2.3

The circulating nurse should identify the procedure performed, the drains (if used), and the need for blood products and blood salvage.

UNFOLDING SCENARIO 2.1D

Alert the anesthesiologist and page the surgeon back to the OR suite. The patient is showing signs of hypervolemia.

UNFOLDING SCENARIO 2.2A

Assess the patient's range of motion related to positioning in lithotomy. Confer with the surgeon and the anesthesiologist on the patient's refusal of blood products. Consider the use of cell salvage.

UNFOLDING SCENARIO 2.2B

- Off the field: Call for the emergency cart and blood salvage device. Call for massive transfusion equipment and products if there is a trauma or massive hemorrhage. Check the suction and be sure that it is operational and that there are multiple empty canisters ready. Ensure that there is warm sterile saline to dispense to the surgical field.
- On the field: Anticipate the surgeon's needs. Monitor the use of sponges or towels and be sure that what was placed in the cavity is removed. Note the canister volume during the transition. If normal saline irrigation is used, take the added volume into account in the suction canister volume when anesthesia wants to know how much blood has been lost. Prepare the room to convert to a fully open procedure. Rapidly provide instrumentation, sutures, and stapling devices as requested by the surgeon.

UNFOLDING SCENARIO 2.2C

- Assist anesthesia personnel in the appropriate laboratory specimen acquisition (i.e., type, screen, and cross) and call the lab personnel to advise that a stat result is needed.
- Follow facility policy and procedure associated with critical lab procurement and transport of the blood specimens to the laboratory.
- Provide assistive service to the surgeon and other personnel at the sterile field.

CHAPTER 3
UNFOLDING SCENARIO 3A

Assessment of the documentation associated with the surgery is required, including history and physical, laboratory and diagnostic results, surgical consent, and anesthesia consent.

POP QUIZ 3.1

Outcome statement: The patient is free from signs and symptoms of electrical injury.

UNFOLDING SCENARIO 3B

The following nursing diagnoses would be considered for this patient:

- Acute pain
- Impaired physical mobility
- Risk for ineffective tissue perfusion
- Risk for infection

POP QUIZ 3.2

PNDS is integrated through perioperative documentation to:

1. Detect the risks associated with patient care.
2. Identify deficiencies in documentation.
3. Improve how electronic documentation is done through the use of preset fields.
4. Standardize documentation through the use of a universal language.

UNFOLDING SCENARIO 3C

The nurse should plan for and anticipate the need for a large specimen box and confer with the physician on the disposition of the limb. *Note:* Some patients may request to retrieve the limb due to cultural practices.

UNFOLDING SCENARIO 3D

The next action is to complete the surgical count of sponges and sharps used in the procedure.

UNFOLDING SCENARIO 3E

Ensure that the patient's leg is fully cleaned, and a new gown is placed on the patient prior to moving the patient to the bed.

CHAPTER 4

UNFOLDING SCENARIO 4A

The perioperative nurse should ask for the team to pause and perform the time-out process.

UNFOLDING SCENARIO 4B

The perioperative nurse should post the x-rays and MRI images for display. All images and diagnostic results needed for the surgery should be posted where all team members can see without obstruction.

POP QUIZ 4.1

Padding should be placed to support the occiput, scapulae, arms, elbows, thoracic vertebrae, sacrum/coccyx, and heels.

UNFOLDING SCENARIO 4C

- Elbows/arms
- Occiput: With a foam or gel headrest
- Operative leg: If in a holder, then it needs to be padded and secured. Check circulation prior to draping.
- Non-operative leg: Securely position as directed by the surgeon and pad the heel.

UNFOLDING SCENARIO 4D

- Ensure that all fluids have been dried from the floor to prevent slip and fall.
- Ensure that the foot of the bed has been elevated and made ready to move the patient's legs back to anatomical position.
- Remain at the side of the bed to assist anesthesia personnel during the patient's emergence from anesthesia.
- Return the safety strap to the patient, if it has been moved during the procedure or following surgical intervention.

POP QUIZ 4.2

The scrub nurse and the circulating nurse should begin a full search of the surgical field and around the field, respectively. While the surgeon continues to work, all of the unnecessary sharps and sponges should be removed from the field. The contents of the kick bucket, the floor, the bottoms of staff shoes, under the furniture, and the room trash (with a magnet if needed) should be evaluated by the circulator. Once those steps are complete, and it is found that the needle is still missing, the surgeon should be notified as radiology may need to be called to assess whether or not the sharp is retained within the body cavity.

POP QUIZ 4.3

The circulating nurse should alert the scrub person that the gown is compromised, and the scrub person should be advised to remove the gown, re-scrub, re-gown, and re-glove.

POP QUIZ 4.4

- Communicate to the team that there is a fire.
- Extinguish the fire, remove the drape, and assess whether there is any additional potential harm to the patient. Once the fire is extinguished, the circulating nurse should replace the damaged drape with a new, sterile one.
- Move the foot pedals to a position that can be seen by the surgeon.

POP QUIZ 4.5

Confirm with the surgeon how the specimen should be sent to pathology and the description of the suture-marked areas.

CHAPTER 5
POP QUIZ 5.1

The nurse should alert the surgeon that assistive personnel cannot be delegated this duty because formal training is required.

UNFOLDING SCENARIO 5A

The circulating nurse should pause and let the visitor know that no one is to move during the time-out. The resident should be asked to move back to the original position.

UNFOLDING SCENARIO 5B

The circulating nurse should immediately go to the resident and assist them into a chair. The nurse should then call the charge nurse to ask for someone to escort the resident out of the OR.

POP QUIZ 5.2

The circulating nurse should ask the healthcare industry representative (HCIR) why they are in the room prior to the patient being draped for surgery. If the representative is assisting the scrub person with the assembly of instrumentation, the nurse may permit them to stay. The nurse should remind the representative to maintain a safe distance from the surgical field to avoid contamination.

POP QUIZ 5.3

The nurse should refrain from opening the contents and notify the manager. In this scenario, the nurse cannot approve the use of the cement because its use would violate facility policy and procedure.

CHAPTER 6

POP QUIZ 6.1

The scrub and circulating nurses should have examined the package integrity, size of the graft, and expiration date prior to dispensation to the surgical field. Cross-monitoring, situational awareness, and effective communication could have prevented the error.

UNFOLDING SCENARIO 6A

Answer 1: The allergies should have been communicated and verified prior to the application of the skin prep. The anesthesia provider and the circulator should have communicated the need for at least one additional person to facilitate positioning of the patient.

Answer 2: The circulating nurse should have confirmed that the strap was secure on both sides and should have communicated that there was pooling of the skin prep solution.

UNFOLDING SCENARIO 6B

The skin assessment postoperatively should be documented. The nurse should also follow facility policy on the filing of an incident report and any notes associated with adverse events or unplanned activities as per facility policy.

POP QUIZ 6.2

The nurse should communicate the findings to the surgeon, who will determine the course of action related to the surgery and document the findings in the patient's health record. The anesthesia team may need to delay induction until the surgeon assesses the patient's heel and makes a decision on whether or not the surgery can be performed.

CHAPTER 7

UNFOLDING SCENARIO 7A

The neutral zone is used to reduce the incidence of sharps injuries.

To protect the patient from microbial contamination, the scrub personnel should remove the knife from the surgical field and safely hand it off to the circulating nurse because it is now contaminated. Next, the scrub personnel should let the circulator know that there is a need for a drape and alert the surgeon that there is a breach in the existing drape. The scrub personnel should also orient the surgeon to the instrument mat and explain that it will be used as the neutral zone for the remainder of the surgical case.

UNFOLDING SCENARIO 7B

The circulating nurse should advise the surgical scrub person who is using alcohol-based hand antisepsis products that this should be performed with the same rigor as the scrubbing performed by using a scrub brush and sponge, attending to each of the four sides of the hands and fingers on both hands.

The circulating nurse should remind the relief nurse to use facility- and U.S. Food and Drug Administration (FDA)-approved hand lotion in the clinical setting to avoid unintentional microbial spread or allergic reactions from patients.

UNFOLDING SCENARIO 7C

The scrub person should follow the facility policy for blood-borne pathogen exposure after notifying the surgeon of the issue. If the scrub person is actively bleeding, it is necessary to confine and contain the bleed away from the sterile field to avoid microbial exposure to the patient and cross-contamination of the sterile field.

UNFOLDING SCENARIO 7D

Because the surgeon has been notified that there is a sterilization issue, and the only other similar tray is in use, the nurse should review the manufacturer's instructions related to IUSS and then proceed with sterilization according to the manufacturer's parameters for steam sterilization.

UNFOLDING SCENARIO 7E

The documentation for IUSS should be complete and include the date, time, instrument(s), cycle parameters, monitoring results, operator information, patient identification, reason for IUSS, and type of cycle used.

All sharps should be removed from the sterile field after the end of the procedure and final count. All sharps should be removed from instrumentation to protect sterile processing staff from sharps injuries. Sharps should be removed using another instrument and not by hand.

POP QUIZ 7.1

Following the facility policies and procedures related to instrument tracking prevents delays and improves communication on the status of instruments in transit.

POP QUIZ 7.2

Assess all areas of the surgical suite for cleanliness before opening sterile contents for the case.

POP QUIZ 7.3

The term for moisture in a pack or tray is "wet pack." The circulating nurse should remove the tray from use before the scrub person reaches for it. The circulating nurse should notify the sterile processing leadership team or designated personnel so that an investigation ensues to determine the cause or causes of the moisture.

CHAPTER 8

POP QUIZ 8.1

The patient is exhibiting signs of anaphylaxis related to the isosulfan blue dye injection. The circulating nurse should call for help and the emergency code cart and then immediately move to the head of the bed to support the patient and the anesthesia personnel. The surgery will come to a pause, a secure airway will be established and confirmed, and the anesthesiologist will order medication to counteract the reaction.

POP QUIZ 8.2

The primary responsibilities of the perioperative circulating nurse in this scenario are as follows:

- Assist the anesthesia personnel as needed.
- Complete a surgical count when it is feasible to do so.
- Open all additional equipment, instruments, sharps, and sponges as requested by the surgeon.
- Provide warmed sterile saline for irrigation of the abdominal cavity.
- Shut off the light source and insufflation machine.
- Turn on the OR lights and room lights.

POP QUIZ 8.3

The perioperative circulating nurse should remain at the head of the bed to provide support for the patient and the anesthesia team as directed by the anesthesiologist of record.

POP QUIZ 8.4

The nurse should cover all cords with facility-approved cord covers and ensure that pathways are not obstructed around the surgical field and within the suite.

POP QUIZ 8.5

The nurse should call for help and ask that the emergency code cart be brought into the suite. The nurse should then begin to open supplies as ordered. The nurse should also coordinate with anesthesia personnel and be prepared to call the blood bank for blood products.

POP QUIZ 8.6

This patient is likely experiencing LAST. The circulating nurse should alert the surgeon that the patient appears confused and that he is bradycardic, call for help to retrieve the rescue kit and emergency code cart, and monitor the airway.

POP QUIZ 8.7

The nurse should call for additional help and the emergency code cart, then begin dilution of dantrolene sodium. The Malignant Hyperthermia Association of the United States (MHAUS) recommends a starting dose of dantrolene at 2.5 mg/kg. Reconstitution of dantrolene will depend upon the brand used. If the facility has a separate malignant hyperthermia (MH) cart, that should be brought into the surgical suite.

POP QUIZ 8.8

Vertical evacuation is necessary as the OR manager has been advised that all patients must be moved to the first floor. The nurse should plan to move the ambulatory patients first. The nurse should always follow the facility fire evacuation plan when moving patients.

POP QUIZ 8.9

The nurse should assist in moving the patient to the supine position to maximize chest compressions and aid with compressions as directed.

POP QUIZ 8.10

The type of trauma is a blunt force. The patient was involved in a motor vehicle accident that resulted in a cervical injury. The circulating nurse should call for a time-out just before the surgeon makes an incision.

CHAPTER 9
POP QUIZ 9.1

3.1 Privacy: Ensure that the patient's body is not needlessly exposed, traffic is minimized, and the doors to the surgical suite are closed.

POP QUIZ 9.2

The organization had mechanisms for reporting the error and completed a root cause analysis (RCA). Additionally, the organization's approach was nonpunitive, evaluating system failures rather than blaming the individual. This scenario describes an organization that employed principles of safety culture.

INDEX

Page entries that appear in italics refer to content in the practice test and practice test answer chapters.